Facilitating the Process of Working Through in Psychotherapy

Facilitating the Process of Working Through in Psychotherapy provides a detailed understanding and de-mystification of the concept of "working through" in dynamic psychotherapy, the most vital but neglected aspect of the therapeutic process.

Just as there are multiple factors responsible for the creation and perpetuation of symptoms and suffering, multiple interventions are frequently required to work through and resolve them. This volume spans topics such as multiple causation, repetition compulsion, and the polarities of experience, while emphasizing the importance of providing a corrective emotional experience, recognizing and repairing ruptures to the alliance and facilitating a positive ending to treatment. Verbatim transcripts of the author's therapy sessions illustrate the factors responsible for working through toward enduring change, and readers are taken through theory, research, and practice.

This book is essential reading for all psychotherapists who are committed to increasing therapeutic effectiveness while enhancing their own personal and professional development.

Patricia Coughlin is a Clinical Psychologist with over 40 years of experience as a therapist and teacher. She is the author of *Maximising Therapeutic Effectiveness in Dynamic Psychotherapy* (Routledge, 2016), *Lives Transformed* (Routledge, 2007), and *Intensive Short Term Dynamic Psychotherapy* (Routledge, 2004). She lectures, teaches, and trains psychotherapists internationally.

Facilitating the Process of Working Through in Psychotherapy

Mastering the Middle Game

Patricia Coughlin

Routledge
Taylor & Francis Group
LONDON AND NEW YORK

Cover image: "Out of the Rubble", 2021, Patricia Coughlin,
www.patriciacoughlinart.com

First published 2023
by Routledge
4 Park Square, Milton Park, Abingdon, Oxon OX14 4RN

and by Routledge
605 Third Avenue, New York, NY 10158

Routledge is an imprint of the Taylor & Francis Group, an informa business

British Library Cataloguing-in-Publication Data
A catalogue record for this book is available from the British Library

ISBN: 978-1-032-05467-4 (hbk)
ISBN: 978-1-032-05468-1 (pbk)
ISBN: 978-1-003-19766-9 (ebk)

DOI: 10.4324/9781003197669

Typeset in Times New Roman
by codeMantra

To the memory of Dr David Malan – the original "iron fist in the velvet glove" – a true English gentleman who was passionate about doing work of depth and significance in the briefest amount of time.

He was convinced that dynamic psychotherapy can be "not merely effective, but uniquely effective", and dedicated his life to the study of psychotherapy in order to prove it. That he and his amazing wife, Jennie, became dear friends has been a true blessing in my life.

Contents

Acknowledgments

This book is the culmination of over 40 years of study and practice in the art and science of dynamic psychotherapy. It couldn't have come to fruition without the help and assistance of many. Jonathan Entis provided the motivation to do the book and encouraged me every step of the way. For reading the manuscript with great care, and providing valuable feedback, I am in debt to Drs Tor Wennerberg, Ron Albucher, Brandon Yarns, and Erin Hall.

I've had extraordinary teachers and supervisors throughout my training and career, most notably Dr David Malan and Dr Habib Davanloo. My colleagues – most of whom have also become dear friends – have been a constant source of support and inspiration and are almost too numerous to mention. Bjorn Elwin, Agneta Bongers, Peter Lillingren, Angela Cooper, Allan Abbass, Allen Kalpin, Jeffrey Magnavita, Jon Frederickson, Diana Fosha, Leigh Mc Cullough, Kristin Osborn, Steven Shapiro, Bruce Ecker, Jonathan Shedler, Susan Fisher, Andrew Ursino, Janet Jaffee, John Rathauser, Robert Neborsky, Josette ten-have de Labije, Jim Schubmehl (my first ISTDP supervisor), David Wolff, Diane Byster, Jody Whitehouse, Martha Stark, and Jennie Malan.

My students and patients teach me something new and valuable every day. Growing with you, and through all of our struggles, has enriched my life without measure.

Finally, my warmest appreciation to Zoe Meyer and Jana Craddock, my editors at Taylor & Francis.

My deepest gratitude to Angel Cardon, who edited and formatted the book in preparation for publication. Her attention to detail and heartfelt commitment to the project were a source of inspiration and support that proved invaluable.

None of this would be possible without my family and friends, who are the very breath to my life. I devote this volume to my three darling grandsons: James, Michael, and Benjamin.

Chapter 1

Working Through

From Insight to Sustained Change

Introduction

In therapy, as in life, it is follow-through that makes all the difference between success and failure; between those who live full and successful lives and those who are a mere flash in the pan. While we all seem to long for the sudden insight that irrevocably alters everything, rendering change effortless, the fact is most enduring change involves focus, determination, and persistence. It also involves the courage to take risks and tolerate anxiety for growth. Such a process is not for the fainthearted. This is as true for the therapist as it is for the patient.

Why write (or read) a book on the process of working through? While the working through phase of therapy is considered the most important in determining the outcome, it is also the most neglected in our field (Aron, 1991; Giovachini, 1975; Wachtel, 2011). In fact, there has not been a single published text devoted to this crucial process. The present volume is an attempt to fill in the gap in order to elucidate and expand upon the various therapeutic processes required to translate emotional insight into enduring change.

Research and clinical experience suggest that neither intellectual insight nor emotional catharsis alone is sufficient to promote deep and lasting change in symptoms and character disturbances. Change is a process, not a singular event. The work is multifaceted and requires us to help patients experience the feelings, wishes, and fantasies they have avoided; face painful and difficult truths; consolidate insights into a solid and coherent sense of self; examine distorted and pathological beliefs; and clearly understand the ways in which their internal conflicts have been played out in relationship to others. The process through which defenses break down, anxiety-provoking feelings are faced and experienced, and insight is consolidated in such a way that enduring change is achieved has been termed "working through."

Working through and resolving the patient's core conflicts, such that he is free from suffering and able to create a meaningful and fulfilling life, is an ambitious goal and not one shared by all therapists. Some are content to reduce or eliminate symptoms or simply produce behavioral change.

DOI: 10.4324/9781003197669-1

If that is the case, this book is probably not for you. However, if you strive to become an expert in your field, achieving better and more consistent results than average, a willingness to push yourself and your patients to achieve ambitious goals seems to be required (Wampold et al., 2017). Embracing such goals is no guarantee of always achieving them, but putting all you've got into the effort, and bolstering that effort with ongoing skill development and knowledge acquisition, is necessary to enhance therapeutic effectiveness. To this end, we will examine the history and evolution of the concept of working through and explore its component parts: the notion of multiple causation, the repetition compulsion, understanding complexity and tolerating uncertainty, balancing the polarities of attachment and autonomy, facilitating a corrective emotional experience, creating and maintaining a strong conscious and unconscious alliance (including dealing with ruptures), attending to meaning and coherence, revising and consolidating an integrated sense of self, and dealing with spiritual matters and concerns as they emerge. Case examples will be used liberally throughout the text in order to illustrate and expand upon the points being made.

What Is Working Through? Evolution of the Concept

In the early days of psychoanalysis, Freud was interested in helping patients face and experience primitive and threatening id impulses; the repression of which he considered the root cause of their symptoms and suffering. Consequently, his initial work involved trying to find ways to bypass resistance in an effort to unearth repressed emotions and the memories with which they were associated. Over time he discovered that such cathartic work was often followed by the "return of the repressed," prompting him to shift his focus from uncovering id impulses to strengthening the ego. In this way, previously unconscious feelings and memories could be tolerated, mastered, and integrated into an ongoing sense of self.

Additionally, Freud noticed that patients were repeating, rather than remembering, their anxiety-provoking and guilt-laden emotional conflicts, both in their current life and in the transference. Breuer found this transfer of unresolved conflicts from the past into the present with the therapist personally distressing and considered it an obstacle to the therapeutic process. In contrast, Freud found that the transference of unresolved conflicts onto the person of the therapist proved the most powerful therapeutic tool in our arsenal, if managed properly. "Only when the resistance is at its height can the analyst, working in common with the patient, discover the repressed instinctual impulses which are feeding the resistance" (Freud, 1914, p. 155). It is just such an experience, in the here and now with the therapist, through which the patient discovers the power of his own unconscious. Through the vehicle of the transference, the forgotten past becomes present with the therapist, where it can be faced, understood, and integrated into a solid sense of self. Playing out these anxiety-provoking impulses and fantasies in one's imagination creates a kind of liminal space between repression and acting out, both of which are destructive. By creating such a healing and therapeutic space, we create a kind of "playground in which it is allowed to expand in almost complete freedom" (Freud, 1914, p. 154). Often, this experience with the therapist, with links to past genetic figures, leads to insight into the original source of his disturbance. Being encouraged to experience and express previously forbidden impulses and fantasies directly toward the therapist, with no untoward consequences, is often profoundly corrective and healing. In this way, the past is resolved in the present.

Late in his life, Freud (1937) came to appreciate the role of the superego's resistance to recovery and healing. He discovered that patients suffered, not only by defending against anxiety-provoking and painful feelings, but also due to an unconscious sense of guilt about these forbidden feelings and wishes, which demands punishment. Furthermore, he discovered that some patients experienced a great deal of secondary gain from their symptoms and were loath to give them up. Both factors must be addressed for lasting change to take place.

Here we begin to understand the notion that multiple factors are often responsible for the creation and maintenance of the patients' disturbance. These include anxiety and resistance to facing one's own primitive impulses, repeating instead of remembering, the unconscious need to suffer, and the secondary gain of illness in alleviating the patient from taking responsibility for his life. The complex and difficult nature of uncovering and removing all factors responsible for the patient's pathology was considered the most arduous, time consuming, and frustrating part of the work. That said, working through, from feeling to de-repression, to insight and change, has been deemed the most important factor in achieving lasting change (Freud, 1914). No wonder many in the field agree that working through is the most difficult and time consuming of our therapeutic tasks. Giovachini (1975) wrote, "the two most enigmatic words in psychoanalysis are 'working through.'"

How Is Working Through Accomplished?

Although much has been written about the opening phase of treatment, as well as the termination phase, there are very few guidelines for maintaining focus, deepening the process, and consolidating change in the mid-phase of treatment. As a result, therapeutic effectiveness often suffers. Like the middle game in chess, there is no play book to guide us. To master the game, you must understand the underlying principles involved so that you can respond both strategically and spontaneously to what arises in the here and now, while keeping your eye on the goal. Just as no two games of chess are ever exactly alike, no two therapies will follow the same trajectory. The successful clinician has a method he is passionate about and skilled in implementing in a structured but flexible manner, taking many factors into account in order to maximize effectiveness (Coughlin, 2017).

Just how is this process of working through accomplished? In "*Remembering, Repeating and Working though*," Freud (1914) suggested that therapy required a necessary division of labor. The therapist's job involved identifying and clarifying the resistances to remembering and experiencing anxiety-provoking emotions. It was then up to the patient to overcome these resistances. In his early work, Freud applied a pressure technique and was quite direct in encouraging patients to take an active role in overcoming their resistances to the therapeutic process. Over time, he became increasingly passive and pessimistic about this process, suggesting that we "bow to the superiority of the superego's resistance." Davanloo (1990) considered this a wrong turn and returned to Freud's early and more active stance in confronting resistance as soon as it appeared.

Therapy is not something that is done to the patient but can only be successful if the patient actively collaborates with the therapist in achieving therapeutic goals. The therapist can guide and encourage the patient in these efforts, but the work of translating these insights into action must be squarely placed in the patient's lap. The patient must, first and foremost, change his conscious attitude toward his illness. "He has usually been content with lamenting it, despising it as nonsensical and under-estimating its importance ..." (Freud, 1914, p. 152). Then, he must find the courage to face "an enemy worthy of his mettle, a piece of his personality, which has solid ground for its existence, and out of which things of value for his future life have to be derived" (Freud, 1914, p. 152).

Again, Freud was referring to multiple factors, including the patient's will and courage to do the work required; the need to understand both the benefit, purpose and cost of symptoms; and, finally, to integrate seemingly disparate and even detestable parts of the self, in order to become whole and live a life of meaning and purpose. This is a multifaceted process involving many steps, which often need to be repeated in order to ensure lasting change. Ultimately, "working through" names a battle to be fought and a labor to be done which the neurosis has, for so long, only served to postpone. This is the struggle within oneself; "it is the labor of *transformation* that makes possible the rejection of the neurotic encumbrance and its symptomatic trappings in favor of a novel and presumably healthier mode of life" (Sedler, 1983, p. 75).

To achieve such ambitious therapeutic goals, "It is evident that greater, not less, knowledge of the manifold intricacies of human behavior is necessary before one can acquire the skill in finding for each individual, the most suitable and economical form of treatment" (Alexander & French, 1946). In the end, they found, "Re-experiencing the old, unsettled conflict, but with a new ending, was the secret of every penetrating therapeutic result." Furthermore, "Only the actual experience of a new solution, in the transference or the everyday life of the patient, gives the patient the conviction that a new solution is possible, and induces him to give up the old neurotic pattern." In this sense, then, the patient must *live through*, and not simply *work through*, the old conflict to a new and more satisfying end. And we, as therapists, must come adept at facilitating just this kind of experience.

Altered Sense of Self

While Freud (1914) emphasized the importance of overcoming resistance, including resolving the transference, in order to uncover and resolve conflicts regarding traumatic memories, subsequent ego psychologists emphasized the need to integrate the previously forgotten memories and repressed feelings into the patient's ongoing sense of self. Along these lines, Wolstein (1982) suggested that it is not enough to work through or overcome the past but to "work toward" a new and expansive future. In the process of renouncing defense and resistance, in order to face and experience conflicted feelings regarding the past, stalled development resumes (Kohut, 1984). Since internal working models of self and others are developed very early in life and often operate out of sight, as a guiding fiction, they must be updated and expanded as new information is assimilated and experience is deepened and expanded.

For example, some who have lost weight and maintained the loss for decades continue to see themselves as "fat," just as those who have been sober for decades may still consider themselves an "addict."

How do behavioral changes result in an alteration in identity and sense of self? To process change on that level, we must revise and reorganize our story or narrative. Whether we are a victim or a hero in that narrative has a huge impact on health, well-being, and overall functioning. It's not just about what one does or doesn't do, but how we see and define ourselves that matters most. This often requires bringing the past into present consciousness and re-evaluating situations and beliefs based on current reality, as opposed to memories from the past. This must also include the employment of current tools and knowledge, rather than outmoded and unexamined beliefs and capacities. It has been said that neurotics are stuck in existential time, with the sense that they are, always have been, and always will be, damaged in some way. As conflicts and problems are addressed and resolved, the meanings associated with them must be reevaluated and revised, along with one's sense of self.

Insight and emotional freedom are not always enough to ensure lasting change. These factors must be integrated into a stable, ongoing sense of self for change to endure. Narratives must be revised, and identities alerted, in order to accommodate a new and expansive sense of self.

Human beings are storytellers and seek to create meaning in their lives. A reflective construction of a new personal meaning is often required to consolidate deep and lasting change. This reflective processing and "symbolization of a client's emotional experience, in the context of salient and personal stories, is viewed as a key intervention strategy that enables clients to meaningfully integrate their narrative and emotional lives …" (Angus et al., 2012, p. 55).

Therapist Factor

The therapist's role in promoting this kind of therapeutic encounter is key. To help patients in this manner, the therapist must be comfortable with the patient's intense and often disturbing feelings and wishes, as well as his own. The therapist with "his technical skill and the transference events are indispensable factors in the overall process" (Loewald, 1960). Research has confirmed the central importance of therapist variables to the outcome. His skill and tenacity, superior meta-cognitive skills, deep domain-specific knowledge, and emotional intelligence exert a far greater impact on the therapeutic outcome than either patient variables or the treatment model employed (Duncan et al., 2009; Kaplowitz, Safran & Muran, 2011).

This speaks to our own development as therapists, including the ability to identify multiple causes of our patient's misery, while tolerating both complexity and uncertainty along the path to resolution. The best therapists have a theory and method they are enthusiastic about and adept at implementing across a wide spectrum of patients. The theory and technique used to guide the work of the author are that of Intensive Short-Term Dynamic Psychotherapy (ISTDP), a multifaceted model of treatment that is garnering increasing empirical evidence as both clinically and cost-effective with a wide variety of patients (Abbass, 2003, 2015; Shedler, 2010). ISTDP has proven effective in treating anxiety, panic disorder, depression (including treatment-resistant depression), personality disorders, and conversion, as well as somatic disorders and unidentified medical symptoms.

ISTDP: A Multi-modal Treatment Model

The therapeutic model used by the author is ISTDP, developed by Habib Davanloo, MD. While a thorough review of the model is beyond the context of this chapter, a quick summary is included. For more detailed information on the method of ISTDP, consult the authors' previous works (Coughlin Della Selva, 1991, 1992, 1993, 1996, 2006, 2007, 2017) as well as those of Davanloo (1978, 1980, 1990, 2000), Abbass (2015), and Fredrickson (2013).

Subsequent to his work with Lindemann on the front lines, with patients who were in a crisis due to external circumstances, Davanloo (1978, 1980) set out to develop a therapeutic technique designed to precipitate an intrapsychic crisis in patients with chronic difficulties. By pressuring the patient to experience feelings he had long been avoiding, and challenging him to abandon defenses rigidly held, he was able to create an intrapsychic crisis that reliably triggered an opening into the unconscious and sped the process of change. Armed with a deep understanding of psychoanalytic theory and a keen intuitive understanding of the unconscious, Davanloo began to experiment with more active and specific techniques. In addition, he videotaped all his sessions in order to track effectiveness. He eventually developed the central dynamic sequence, a structured but flexible method for reliably obtaining ambitious therapeutic goals with a wide range of patients, in a relatively brief period of time (Davanloo, 1978, 1980, 1990, 2000).

When Malan (Davanloo, 1978, 1980) first observed this work on videotape, he was able to see the ways in which Davanloo was using the two triangles to navigate the therapeutic process (Figure 1.1). All of the specific interventions he had developed were integrated into a process of dynamic assessment (which he referred to as a "trial therapy") that was designed to gather specific information about the difficulties to be addressed. These data were then used to formulate, and test out, a hypothesis about the nature of the conflicts responsible for these difficulties. Ultimately, the patient's response to intervention was employed as the primary diagnostic tool and guide to further intervention. This method of assessment was also designed to assess the patient's current capacity to engage in this intensive form of treatment.

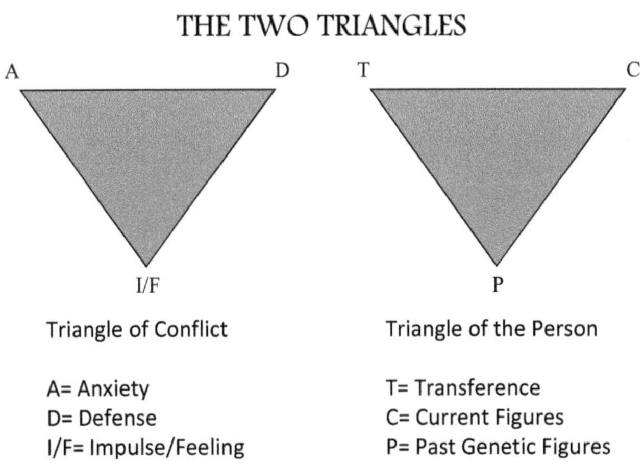

Figure 1.1 The Two Triangles.

Phase I: Inquiry

Davanloo (1978, 1980, 1990) advocated a phenomenological approach to inquiry, in which a specific and detailed examination of the patient's presenting problems is the initial focus. Understanding the nature, history, and severity of the problems to be addressed is step one in the process. This includes an examination of the situations and triggers in which symptoms and presenting problems arise, with a particular emphasis on the precipitating incident motivating the patient to seek treatment.

Right from the start, we must be attentive to the creation of a therapeutic alliance. At this phase of the work, we attempt to achieve agreement about the problems and goals for therapy. Agreement on the therapeutic task, another essential element in the creation of a conscious therapeutic alliance, often takes place later in the process, once defenses have been relinquished. It should be noted that, during the opening phase of inquiry, only defenses that interfere with the process of obtaining this vital information are addressed. When defenses, such as vagueness, externalization, or defiance, prevent the phase of inquiry from taking place in any meaningful way, the process must move to phase II, defense work.

Phase II: Defense Work

Davanloo (1990) developed operational definitions of many dynamic concepts and processes, including that of defense work. This process involves (1) the identification and (2) clarification of defenses, as well as (3) an examination of costs and benefits of the defenses in question. It is essential that the patient is helped to see that his symptoms and presenting problems are created and/or exacerbated by the habitual use of defenses. Once he sees clearly that his defensive avoidance of his true feelings is the engine perpetuating his difficulties, and is able to enumerate the negative consequences of such avoidance, he is put at choice – to continue to suffer or face his true feelings in order to heal and obtain his freedom from suffering.

Defense work often evokes strong feelings in the patient, either grief over the cost of his defenses or anger toward the therapist for pointing them out. Again, the patient is put at choice – to face or avoid the feelings coming up in the here and now.

Assessment and Regulation of Anxiety

One of the most common mistakes therapists make is keeping anxiety too low for change to take place. As soon as the patient becomes uncomfortable, they pull back. In contrast, Davanloo (personal communication, 1988–1991) encouraged us to move in and focus on the conflicts and feelings triggering anxiety. His method has been based on Freud's second theory of anxiety, suggesting that anxiety is a signal, alerting the therapist to an area of pain and distress that needs to be examined.

Davanloo (1990) identified three channels of anxiety, which are highly diagnostic. When patients channel anxiety into their voluntary striated muscle, it indicates good capacity and suggests that threatening feelings, impulses, and fantasies are close to the surface, where they can be safely uncovered. Muscle tension, sighing respiration, and hand clenching are cardinal signs of striated muscle anxiety and are a "green light," indicating that the patient is activated and ready to work. There is also neuroscientific evidence that moderate levels of anxiety are essential to brain and behavior change in adults. When anxiety is too low, change does not take place. If anxiety is too high and is overwhelming the system, therapeutic change cannot take place. Working in the patient's optimal zone of anxiety tolerance is required to proceed safely but effectively toward therapeutic change.

We expect patients to be anxious when consulting a therapist and must pay attention to signs of anxiety activation in the body. If not in evidence, we must explore further to determine where the anxiety is going. In such cases, anxiety is either being channeled into the smooth muscle (with headaches, irritable bowel syndrome, and other somatic markers of anxiety) or cognitive/perceptual disruption (e.g. confusion, dissociation, blurry vision, and ringing in the ears). Alternatively, the patient may be detached and uninvolved in the process, perhaps even in the office against his will. Determining whether high and unregulated anxiety or defense and resistance are responsible for this lack of muscle activation is essential in finding the appropriate intervention for each patient – either downregulating anxiety or addressing defenses.

Phase III: Breakthrough of Feelings

When feelings arise, either toward the therapist, or someone in the patient's current life with whom the presenting difficulties are manifest, the therapist exerts pressure on the patient to experience these feelings directly and viscerally, in the here and now. This is a three-pronged process including (1) a clear declaration of feeling toward a specific individual, (2) the physiological activation and experience of the feeling in question, and (3) mobilization of the impulse or action tendency accompanying the stated feeling. Davanloo (1990) found that the visceral experience of previously avoided feelings, especially in the transference, was the key to a rapid opening or unlocking of the unconscious, followed by a de-repression of memories, dreams, and associations shedding light on the origin of the patient's conflicts.

This process seems to unleash an inner healing force in the patient that Davanloo has referred to as the *unconscious therapeutic alliance* (UTA). Without conscious awareness or intention, the patient's unconscious provides information to the therapist, helping her understand the nature and source of the difficulties. This phenomenon can manifest in the form of slips of the tongue, sudden memories, and associations or images emerging from the unconscious which shed light on the origin of the patient's conflicts. Managing the twin forces of alliance and resistance, both conscious and unconscious, must remain in the forefront of the therapist's attention throughout treatment.

Once the patient is clear about what he is feeling toward whom, is experiencing the physiological activation characteristic of that emotion, and shows evidence of mobilization of impulse (hands in fists, kicking foot, etc.), Davanloo advocated the use of visualization to "portrait" the forbidden impulses being experienced. Internalizing these impulses or acting them out are both highly destructive defenses. In contrast, using one's imagination to face anxiety-provoking and guilt-laden feelings and impulses, without anyone getting hurt, is the task during this phase of the treatment. Once the patient faces their ultimately mixed feelings (toward the therapist or person in their current life being focused upon), a transfer of images, in which an attachment figure from the past (whom the current person has come to represent) appears spontaneously, often takes place. This highly charged emotional experience is the trigger unlocking the unconscious, paving the way to healing.

Phase IV: De-repression and Interpretation

Links between the emotional conflicts being experienced in the patient's current life (C), in the transference situation (T), and the past (P) are made at this point, often by the patient himself. At this juncture, a meaningful examination of the past is possible. With defenses out of operation, and the alliance in full command, memories associated with the original source of the patient's core conflicts are revealed in an undisguised fashion. Feelings and behavior that had previously bewildered the patient now begin to make sense. It seems as if there is coherence in the unconscious (Ecker et al., 2012), providing clear links between the unresolved past and the patient's current suffering.

When all goes well, and the patient is capable of tolerating their own unconscious feelings and memories, the central dynamic sequence can be completed in the initial trial therapy (typically three hours in length). Sometimes this is all that is required. In fact, research suggests that as many as one-third of our patients resolve the conflicts responsible for their presenting complaints in this initial encounter. In these cases, no further treatment is required (Abbass, Joffres & Ogrondniczuk, 2008; Abbass et al., 2014, 2017; Abbass & Schubiner, 2018; Shedler, 2010). More commonly, additional therapy is necessary but gets off to a strong start with this extended initial session, as both motivation and alliance are greatly enhanced via this process.

To remove bias, Davanloo (personal communication, 1988–1991) has urged therapists to conduct this extended initial session blind to the patient's difficulties and psychiatric history. Rather than gather data on the phone, or read other's reports prior to seeing the patient, he suggested we see him with fresh eyes. In this way, we can assess the patient's ability to respond therapeutically to intervention in the here and now, without prejudice or preconceived notions on our part.

Davanloo, like many of the most effective therapists who have been studied (Wampold, 2001; Wampold & Imel, 2015), was very ambitious. His therapeutic goals included the full resolution of the patient's conflicts and difficulties, with each symptom and pathological defense replaced with something healthy. Furthermore, he challenged himself and his patients to tolerate anxiety for growth and to persist, rather than give up, when difficulties in the process arose.

While ISTDP is a structured and flexible method of dynamic psychotherapy, many of the interventions can be utilized and integrated into other approaches. Each phase of the central dynamic sequence is supported by research, which has associated each factor with a positive outcome in psychotherapy (Coughlin, 2017).

The Patient's View

So far, we have explored the therapist's view of the process of working through, but what is corrective or therapeutic about therapy from the patient's point of view? Heatherington and colleagues (2012) studied this question and asked patients (1) *what* had changed as the result of therapy and (2) *how* that change had been accomplished. The majority of patients (65%) who had received cognitive behavioral, humanistic, or psychodynamic psychotherapy mentioned "new experiential awareness" as a key factor in the change process. By experiencing feelings they had been avoiding, patients came to a new and deeper understanding of themselves and their relationships, as well as the meaning and significance of their symptoms and presenting problems. Insight and self-awareness were cited as the most important factors in the attainment of therapeutic goals (this was also confirmed by Pennebaker, 1997). Of interest, these therapeutic goals were viewed as something achieved by the patient himself, as opposed to having been provided by the therapist. Other research underscores the importance of the patient viewing change as the consequence of their own efforts, as opposed to those of the therapist (Ecker et al., 2012; Pennebaker, 1997; Piliero, 2004). That said, these patients mentioned therapist focus, engagement, encouragement, and support as crucial in facilitating their newfound awareness. These new affective experiences led to a refreshed and revised perspective on themselves, their relationships, and the connection between past and present, creating a kind of upward trajectory of positive change. In addition, since they had attributed therapeutic gains to their own efforts, the patient's sense of mastery and competence was also enhanced – another factor associated with lasting change (Weinberger, 1995).

The aforementioned studies confirm the findings of other research that underscores the need to develop insight and a new level of self-understanding in order to develop deep and transformational change. Once again, the question is, what therapeutic action facilitated such insight? In a study by McAleavey and Castonguay (2013), specific therapeutic interventions associated with patient insights were explored. Contrary to expectation, they found that therapists who were focused and directive were more successful in facilitating insight than those who promoted open exploration. This direct focus on areas of difficulty tended to evoke strong feelings that had previously been avoided. Alexander and French (1946) discovered that such feelings tended to promote insight, rather than the other way around (the idea that the correct interpretation would lead to feeling). Subsequent research has validated this finding (Messer & McWilliams, 2007; Raingruber, 2000).

Insight, defined as novel cognitive and emotional connections, has been validated as a common factor in all successful psychotherapy. However, insight was typically not achieved by common factors alone (McAleavey & Castonguay, 2013). Those therapists who directed their focus on specific areas of distress, within an atmosphere rich with common factors, were most highly successful in promoting positive change. Focusing on the transference pattern of behavior was particularly transformative for patients with poor levels of object relations (Johansson et al., 2010; Piper et al., 1991). Importantly, this kind of direct focus was not effective in the absence of common factors. These results reinforce those by McCarthy (2009) and colleagues on the importance of combining common and specific factors in effective psychotherapy.

Summary

In this first chapter of the book, we have started our examination of the concept of working through with a general overview of the topic, as well as exploring ways in which such a vital process can be facilitated, from both the therapist's and patient's point of view. In the second chapter, we will focus on the necessity of working through from the very first encounter with the patient. Herein, it is suggested that working through is an ongoing process, to be facilitated in each session, rather than a separate phase of the therapy. In Chapter 3, we will discuss the issue of complexity and multiple causation as it relates to our understanding of psychopathology and process of healing. The notion of a repetition compulsion will be elucidated in Chapter 4. In Chapter 5, we will explore the theme of rupture and repair in the therapeutic relationship, while in Chapter 6, we will understand the central importance of a corrective emotional experience. The balance between the innate drives to attach and to achieve autonomy and self-definition will be the focus of Chapter 7. In the final chapter, ways in which we can facilitate a positive ending to therapy, in order to achieve a good goodbye and consolidate therapeutic gains, will be reviewed. In each chapter, verbatim transcripts from videotaped treatments conducted by the author will be used to illustrate the points being made.

Chapter 2

Working Through from the Start

The Central Importance of the Initial Encounter

Sullivan asserted that skill in psychotherapy consists in doing as much with as little as possible. Never is that statement more apt than during the initial consultation. Patients are rarely more anxious, distressed, and hopeful – in other words, more intensely conflicted – than when they first arrive at the therapist's office. Taking advantage of this kind of activation, and striking while the iron is hot, is a crucial therapeutic skill to hone. All too often this window of opportunity is squandered, and the patient never returns.

While most therapists are trained to make descriptive diagnoses (like those contained in the DSM V), and are encouraged to focus on developmental history, neither factor has proven to have much predictive value (Craddock & Owen, 2010). Back in the 1960s, Malan and his colleagues at the Tavistock Clinic in London (Malan, 1963, 1976) discovered that response to a trial interpretation was far more predictive of a positive outcome in short-term dynamic psychotherapy than history or diagnosis. Much to their surprise, they discovered that the most profound therapeutic changes occurred in patients with chronic difficulties in many areas of functioning. The key to success was a "radical" technique in which the therapist took up negative feelings and reactions in the transference as soon as they appeared. In addition, the most effective therapists were experts at spotting patterns. In particular, they were able to see the patient's current crisis as the most recent iteration of a repetitive conflict, with its origins in the past. The patient's ability to respond *emotionally* to such an interpretation, linking their current problems with unresolved conflicts from the past, proved highly prognostic.

Davanloo (1990) expanded upon the notion of "response to interpretation" and created the structure for a "trial therapy," in which all active elements of his treatment approach are applied in an extended initial evaluation, typically three hours in length (Coughlin, 2017; Davanloo, 1990; Malan & Coughlin Della Selva, 2007). The patient's response to each intervention is employed as the primary diagnostic tool and guide to intervention. Assessing the patient's capacity to respond in a therapeutic manner in real time appears to be the most accurate and timely data upon which to make clinical decisions.

DOI: 10.4324/9781003197669-2

The Central Dynamic Sequence in ISTDP

Davanloo (1978, 1980) took a scientific approach to psychotherapy, treating each case as an N = 1 study. He gathered specific data about the nature, history, and severity of the presenting problems in order to develop a hypothesis about the unconscious conflicts responsible for the patient's difficulties. He tested out his hypothesis with a variety of interventions, using the patient's response to intervention in order to confirm, refute, or reconstruct his case conceptualization. All cases were videotaped, studied, and shared with patients, in order to determine the factors responsible for therapeutic change. After experimenting in this manner for years, Davanloo developed a method of assessment and intervention he referred to as *The Central Dynamic Sequence.* These steps include a nuanced and multi-modal approach to the process. Unlike many, Davanloo (1978, 1980, 1990) did not advocate beginning the process of assessment with an examination of the past. Rather, he suggested we begin with the patient's current difficulties, as this is where their motivation lies. In addition, since defenses are almost always in place at the start of therapy, and defenses distort memories, he urged us to postpone an examination of the past once the unconscious is open and fluid. He also suggested that we enter the initial evaluation blind to the patient's problems and history so that we can assess him in real time rather than beginning with preconceived notions.

The wisdom of such an approach was made clear to me early in my training with Davanloo. A middle-aged woman contacted me by phone to set up an initial evaluation. She seemed eager to fill me in on her life story but, following Davanloo's suggestion, I said, "Let's wait until you arrive, and we'll go into all this in depth." During the trial therapy, I learned that this woman had suffered from both migraine headaches and periods of frequent dissociation since childhood, a childhood marred by extensive physical and sexual abuse (this case, "The Dissociative Woman," was outlined in detail in my first book). Had I known this history ahead of time, I would have assumed that she would be quite fragile and would require long-term, supportive therapy. In fact, she proved highly responsive and extremely resilient. We were able to understand the current crisis in light of unresolved feelings from the past, which were activated and processed in the very first session. Her entire treatment only lasted 14 sessions, something I never would have imagined possible given her history. The result of our work included a resolution of her conflicts, the complete removal of debilitating symptoms, and a resumption of development that had been arrested for years. At ten-year follow-up, she was nearly unrecognizable. In fact, she looked younger and more vital than she had appeared during our initial meeting a decade earlier. As is typical in patients who respond well to Intensive Short-Term Dynamic Psychotherapy (ISTDP), she was better and stronger than at termination with no further treatment (Abbass, 2003; Abbass, Town & Driessen, 2012; Shedler, 2010).

This case illustrates many key points, in particular, the need to evaluate patients in real time, scheduling enough time to administer the central dynamic sequence in the first contact with the patient, and facilitating a therapeutic experience in the first contact. Doing so strengthens the conscious and unconscious alliance and accelerates the process of change.

While we typically think of working through as taking place during the mid-phase of therapy, this process can, and often does, take place during each session, including the initial contact. When we think of "working through" as the deep understanding of one's inner life, appearing after the breakdown of defenses and the actual experience of the feelings and emotions that had been previously avoided, we begin to understand that this process can and must take place in each session.

Evidence suggests that therapists who conduct extensive initial sessions tend to get superior results to those who only schedule an hour-long session for the first contact (Abbass, Joffres & Ogrondniczuk, 2008). Rather than simply taking a developmental history, we need time to understand the patient's current difficulties and their precipitants in some depth, in order to identify the defenses that are causing or exacerbating these problems, to facilitate the experience of feelings that have been avoided, and to discover the driving force of the patient's symptoms and suffering. In so doing, we are likely to facilitate a therapeutic experience during the first encounter, intensifying and accelerating the entire therapeutic process.

When we learn to use the initial evaluation as a therapeutic instrument, deep and lasting change can be achieved in a brief period of time. Taking the time and learning to implement a systematic but flexible dynamic evaluation is essential in achieving these kinds of results. Given the tremendous need for mental health services in this country, and around the world, and the lack of availability of skilled help to aid those who are suffering, learning to be as efficient and effective as possible is more urgent than ever.

One of the most robust findings regarding a positive and rapid response to treatment is when the patient is in the midst of a crisis. Almost by definition, a crisis is precipitated by events that evoke such intense and conflictual feelings that the patient's typical defenses break down, resulting in symptoms and presenting difficulties. The first research on the effectiveness of short-term dynamic psychotherapy underscored this fact (Malan, 1963). The combination of a patient in crisis with a highly skilled therapist who is able to understand the crisis as the most recent example of a recurrent conflict, was found to be highly predictive of positive outcomes in short-term dynamic psychotherapy (Malan, 1976, 1979).

Davanloo (1990) went a step further and developed a method designed to precipitate a crisis in patients who are cemented in their character difficulties, greatly expanding the number of patients we can help in a relatively brief period of time. This kind of intrapsychic crisis is created when the patient is confronted with the cost of his defenses and challenged to give them up in favor of facing his feelings directly in order to heal and reclaim his emotional freedom.

Therapy Completed in the Initial Evaluation

The following case was completed in a four-hour initial consultation. The patient was seen for an initial three-hour session, with a one-hour follow-up the next day. We were able to discover the conflicts responsible for the patient's lifelong difficulties, and work them through in such a way that he was freed from suffering and able to move forward and achieve his goals. Material gathered at a three-year follow-up confirmed that he was better than ever. In other words, all symptoms and pathological defenses had been replaced with something healthy, allowing his development to resume unimpeded. Given that this man had sought out therapy a number of times previously and had not achieved therapeutic benefits, it appeared that this approach (and this therapist) was far more effective for him than other methods (and/or other therapists) had been.

Man in a Cage

TH: *Tell me why you're here and how I can help?*

PT: *I'm here to (sigh) – oh, yeah, this is the question I am anxious about or dreading, since I made the appointment, I guess. So, I thought I tried to feel about it and I guess (sigh) guilt, um … I feel caged or not free. I don't feel free to be myself (sigh), so guilt, shame, and where that comes from.*

TH: *And what is it all about? You don't really know what it's about, but you're locked in it? For how long would you say?*

PT: *That's a really scary question, I think. Cause I don't know … maybe since I was 10 – probably before. I'm not sure. Just afraid of what I will find – a monster or something.*

TH: *This has been going on for a long time. What brings you right now?*

It is essential that we discover the CURRENT precipitant to the patient's suffering, even if it has been lifelong. Why is the patient seeking help now? Is it his will to engage in a therapeutic process or are they caving in under pressure from others? Discovering the source of suffering and motivation is a central task of the initial inquiry and all too often missed or neglected.

PT: *A while ago, I went into a serious depression. Stuff was happening. My mother's life was tanking. We were trying to have a second baby by IVF. My work was very difficult. I just broke down and got hyper anxious for months. I pondered suicide, but of course I didn't.*

TH: *It was so unbearable?*

PT: *It was unbearable, so I need to tell you this – I asked for a sick leave and was offered therapy and I went to a consultation and this person ... an ISTDP therapist...I was so low that I couldn't ... but ...*

TH: *What were you going to say?*

PT: *He overran me. I felt a bit trampled on. I didn't know what happened. I tried to figure it out. After the first session, I was more broken than before.*

This is a danger that all therapists must be careful to avoid – taking over and dominating the interaction, rather than highlighting the cost of the patient's subservience and compliance.

TH: *That's terrible.*

PT: *Yeah, that was terrible, actually. And I don't know if we ever sorted that out. No, there was a problem with trust. Something was off and since then I've had this in mind to come to see you.*

TH: *Why me? You had one bad experience but wanted to try again, so why come here?*

PT: *I wanted to come East for a sabbatical, so I thought, "While I'm there I'll go see someone there." I wrote an email and never imagined I would hear back. I thought, "This will never happen." But you responded right away.*

While the patient initially tied his anxiety to a fear of looking within (and possibly discovering "a monster"), he also revealed conflicting feelings about opening up to the therapist and engaging in an intimate therapeutic relationship, having had a bad experience with a previous therapist. In this case, both interpersonal and intrapsychic conflicts were present from the start and needed to be addressed. When a patient is fending off authentic contact with the therapist, no treatment, no matter how effective, will be of use. Defenses against closeness and opening up to the therapist must always be our first priority.

It became clear that the "cage" this patient complained of was one he had created to keep himself from opening up and being close with others, for fear of being misunderstood or betrayed yet again (and feeling all his feelings about that!). At the same time, the fact that he revealed all this so openly was a sign that both his conscious and unconscious alliances were quite strong from the start. This created an opportunity to ally with his motivation and help him overcome his resistance so that progress could be made rapidly.

Identifying Defenses against Emotional Closeness in the Transference

TH: *It's interesting, when I talk, you look at me and pay attention, but when you talk, you look away and disconnect. Are you aware of that? You don't look at me when you speak to me.*

PT: *(Starts to cry) That happens all the time.* (Response to intervention suggests this is where the money is right now. He may, in fact, be afraid to face his own truth, but the mixed feelings coming up in transference are more palpable). *Yes, yes, like on the plane coming here. I sat next to this really, really nice guy and he was looking intensely at me, but I had to look away, I couldn't bear it.* (This new information confirms the primacy of defenses against closeness).

TH: *So you know you are anxious and avoiding, but what are you feeling?*

PT: *Can I trust them?*

TH: *Those are some thoughts. You are aware of anxiety, thoughts about trust, and then creating distance – but not what the feelings are … that is a blind spot.*

PT: *That is a blind spot. I've never gone into that, but the same thing happened when I met a colleague in NY for drinks and the same thing happened. He's this intense guy. I'm, ah … This wears me out.*

TH: *What? The anxiety?*

PT: *Not being in the present.* (Starting to turn on the defense as he experiences the cost.)

TH: *Sure, and, in so doing, you deprive yourself of connection and being seen and understood.*

PT: *Yeah (tears up) that's probably – yeah. Yeah. You are hitting a sore spot when you say that, because that is what it's about, but I don't know what feeling that is.*

TH: *There's a lot of pain it looks like.*

PT: *Yes! Yeah.*

TH: *Can we just look at that? There is a lot of pain around this issue of wanting to be seen and understood but part of you is terrified and keeping a distance and it's very painful for you.*

PT: *It is.*

TH: *And lonely I would think.*

PT: *Yes, lonely. Very lonely. Lonely and afraid. (crying).*

While the patient did not initially present with difficulties regarding close relationships, these problems emerged as the therapist pointed out the transference pattern of behavior. We can only gauge the level of resistance by tracking the patient's response to interventions involving the identification of defenses. In this case, the patient was highly responsive to the therapist's observations about his tendency to create emotional distance with her, suggesting a high level of motivation and a relatively low level of resistance. This led to a frank acknowledgment of this problem in his life, with several recent and specific examples. These responses to intervention – the fact that he was able to see how defenses against closeness were operating in his life, understood their function, and experienced grief over their cost – suggested that his defenses were becoming dystonic. That set the stage for highlighting and intensifying this core conflict.

TH: *So this is a dilemma because on the one hand, if you can avoid contact, the anxiety goes down some* (articulating the benefit of the defense).

PT: *To a certain point.*

TH: *But then you're alone with these feelings. We can see that you're here but not here – keeping a certain distance, not able to look at me when you're talking. What is the consequence of that? First of all, how will you know if I am really available and attentive, and you are keeping yourself alone with these painful feelings?*

PT: *Yes! Yeah. (crying) Yeah … It makes me feel a flicker of anger.*

TH: *And you can feel that coming here. How do you feel that anger toward me?*

PT: *Towards you? It's probably someone from the past, like Mom or Dad. This story pops up and I have to tell – I don't have to, but I'm going to tell you, and I'm going to try and look at you as I tell it.* (This statement suggests that change is already happening – the patient catches defense in operation and takes a stand against it, going in a healthy direction). *Now my Mom has Alzheimer's disease. This was what was happening the time when I got depressed, but that's not it. We had a Christmas party. My Mom and Dad are divorced, but he's there because he's part of the family. My aunt was there, and she said, "You had colic as a baby and cried all the time and we were going to babysit you." This was part of a family talk – like a funny … people are … So, anyway, she said, "You were crying and crying", and I thought, "what are we going to do about this" and your parent's said, "just let him cry", but my aunt said, "I couldn't do that" (crying). She said, "I had to take you up in my arms" and I felt, I just felt this fury – this fury at my parents to leave me alone crying – you bastards! (sobbing). That's the first time I've heard about that, and it was in a semi-formal setting so what could I say? I said, "at least someone was nice to the baby. Thanks Aunt." My father was like, "Oh" and pulled back, like he knew it wasn't right.*

As we examined the patient's conflict about opening up with me and others (T-C link), a very meaningful link was made to the source of this conflict, involving unresolved feelings from the past with his parents. The focus on his conflict regarding closeness in the transference boosted both the conscious and unconscious alliances, which shed light on the origin of his difficulties. He was highly emotionally engaged and made meaningful connections between painful and anxiety-provoking feelings and the memories with which they were associated. Research suggests that this kind of connection of emotional and cognitive material, often at the heart of working through, is highly associated with positive outcomes in psychotherapy (Malan, 1976; Malan & Coughlin Della Selva, 2007).

Defenses distort relationships and undermine the development of a collaborative therapeutic alliance. When patients abandon defenses against closeness, and risk being open and emotionally available, the alliance is strengthened and a new, healthy way of relating begins. Research suggests that some therapists are far more effective than others in establishing and maintaining an alliance, especially with difficult and resistant patients (Baldwin, Wampold & Imel, 2007; Del Re et al., 2012; Orlinsky, Grawe & Parks, 1994). Research (Ackerman & Hilsenroth, 2003; Town et al., 2012) suggests that the therapist's ability to elicit affective experience and expression creates stronger alliances and, consequently, better outcomes. Therapists who have high levels of emotional intelligence seem to be more adept at creating a strong alliance with a wide group of patients than their less attuned colleagues (Kaplowitz, Safran & Muran, 2011; Muran, Safran & Eubanks-Carter, 2010). This suggests we must do our own personal work so that we can be an open and engaging presence and not have our own defenses against emotional closeness getting in the way.

Results from a process study on change moments in therapy (Valdes et al., 2010) indicate that the most effective therapists are skillful at deepening and expanding the feelings reported by the patient, rather than those introduced by the therapist. Moreover, research (Buchheim et al., 2012) underscores the need to integrate the affective and cognitive experience. Neither feelings nor cognitive insight alone are sufficient to work through and resolve the patient's conflicts (Stalikas & Fitzpatrick, 1995; Watson, 1996). In fact, such integration seems to lead to neurobiological changes in the neural pathways associated with emotional reactivity and control.

TH: *That was just this past Christmas, so you already had children of your own. So you know what it is to have babies.*

PT: *My daughter had colic, but we carried her around for 3 months, no sleep or anything (crying). That's what you do to a baby, you pick it up and caress it and show it love even though it's … that's what you do!* (Now another link is made between past and present – his relationship to his father and BEING a father.)

TH: *It's incredibly painful and you're absolutely furious with both of them. Who comes first? You mentioned your father. Is it him or?*

PT: *Yes.*

TH: *How do you feel this anger toward your father that he just left you to cry?*

PT: *Yes, it's coming up. It starts and then it stops.*

TH: *Where do you feel that anger in your body?*

PT: *Sigh. It's, it's I can't imagine it now. Yeah. I go flat.*

TH: *Something about facing the rage toward him is threatening so you flatten yourself instead. You protect him – not just there, but even here. Where does it go and what happens to that anger?*

PT: *I guess it goes back to me.*

TH: *You guess? Even now you kind of slump down, do you feel that? You go heavy or weak or what?*

PT: *Yeah, sort of indifferent.*

TH: *You numb out and detach and then eventually get depressed, like that time.*

PT: *Well, I had to.*

In this vignette, we examined specific defenses (going flat and depressed) against a specific feeling (anger), a core conflict for him. Once again, the therapist needed to help the patient see that his reliance on defenses was directly responsible for his symptomatic suffering. This increased his motivation to relinquish them.

TH: *OK – you said one 5 years ago, trying for the second child. Why did you have to do IVF?*
PT: *My wife has endometriosis. That was when my wife, wait, one of the last in vitro* [3 times] *and didn't work or maybe ... my wife got pregnant, and she aborted.*
TH: *Spontaneously?*
PT: *Yeah (sigh). What I think is that I didn't really want to do all those mother fuckers.*

This material suggested that the patient's defenses against his anger toward his wife were likely responsible for the depression. A reference to his mother indicated a possible link there as well. Those issues were explored, so that these hypotheses could be supported, revised, or abandoned. The use of the phrase "mother fuckers" suggests the possibility of some sort of fusion of sexual and aggressive impulses. It was not clear who this was referring to – women or babies.

TH: *A huh. So who wanted that?*
PT: *My wife.*
TH: *Again, there is a lot of feeling coming up and it looks like anger, in this relation.*
PT: *Yes! Yes. That's not easy to talk about.*
TH: *But you liven up – notice the change when you are honest about that.*
PT: *When we got together, she was older than me and she got pregnant, but that was too early, so we had an abortion. Then she started to get symptoms and the doctor said you better get going and have babies before this gets worse. I was still young – like 26 – and I wanted to enjoy life and go here and there and then bang – let's get serious and have babies and only have sex when I'm ovulating – oh my god!* (Punches his fist into his opposite hand.)
PT: *Yeah, so can you feel that anger coming up?*
TH: *Yes, that sucks, and my wife knows it sucks but she says, "You agreed to go on this path with me." Yeah, but I didn't agree how long we have to stay on it, and when to say no and stop; so I don't really feel she has taken my feelings or perspective into consideration.*
PT: *Were you clear about it?*
TH: *No, no I wasn't.*
PT: *So this issue of you swallowing your anger. You go flat, passive, and compliant.*

Here a clear link was made between his tendency to go weak, flat, and passive (D) in the face of his anger (I/F) (the triangle of conflict) – initially with his father, and then in relation to his wife (triangle of person). In contrast to the effects of repression, the therapist pointed out how lively he became when he acknowledged his anger.

TH: *Withholding and detached – so you pay a price for swallowing this anger, not only toward your parents and your wife and, interestingly, all around this issue of babies. It's loaded – these feelings about having a baby, wanting a baby, and you being cared for.*
PT: *Yeah.*
TH: *So where should we start? Toward your wife?*
PT: *Yes, I can feel it now.*
TH: *How does it feel inside?*
PT: *Like energy and a spark or something. Whoooo!*
TH: *You get a little anxious about that anger and what it could do, because if it was let loose and it came out of the cage, here with me. What does that anger want to do? So, if that came out at me, because whenever anyone gets close this gets activated, like with the guy in the plane. Wanting to be seen but then all the pain and rage about being left there just comes up. If that came up? What's in your fists there?*
PT: *But when you ask me to show it to you, it goes.*

We worked and reworked the conflict between his feelings of anger, the anxiety that generated, and the cost of his defenses against his anger, both in his life and in the therapeutic process. While there was no obvious anger toward the therapist in view, the fact that he was defending with distancing defenses suggested it might be present. In any case, this process of restructuring defenses is a repetitive and circular process, in which we go around both triangles. This phase of the work was designed to help him turn on the defenses that caused his symptoms and suffering. As defense and resistance were increasingly weakened, the unconscious therapeutic alliance (UTA) was boosted.

In studying the process of therapeutic change, Mergenthaler (2008) identified four levels of emotional and cognitive activation required to work through and resolve the patient's difficulties. These include (1) relaxation, (2) reflecting, (3) experiencing, and (4) connecting. While it is essential to facilitate an emotional experience, and to prompt reflection upon these feelings, the task of "connecting" appears to be most crucial in determining therapeutic success. "Connecting cycles" in which heightened emotional activation is accompanied by reflection, particularly regarding links between the unresolved past and the patient's current difficulties, appears to be the key to deep and lasting change. These deep emotional connections tend to evoke positive emotions which are associated with growth and expansion (Fredrickson, 2010). Furthermore, when the patient makes these connections himself, his sense of self-mastery and competence is greatly enhanced (another factor associated with lasting change). Of interest, these connections seem to be most impactful during the early and middle phase of a therapy session rather than at the end. This is a reminder to start this crucial work as soon as possible in the session, allowing time for the mastery of deeper levels of conflict to take place by mid-session (Grenyar & Luborsky, 1996). In this case, we can see just such connections being made, as well as observing the boost this creates in the alliance.

TH: *And you're also angry.*

PT: *Yes, I have an example. There's a time when I am 9 or 10 and we went to a family gathering. We were driving back home, and my only male cousin was in the car with my dad driving, and now I'm going to look at you* (self-correcting once again). *I need to do that! He was 3–4 years older than me. We got into the garage, and I said something cocky to be cool and Dad elbowed me and said, "Oh you're being tough now, huh?" Derogatory. I'm trying something out with my cousin. I remember being pushed down.*

TH: *That's what he did – put you down – "don't think you can be a man". So what kind of feeling do you have toward him?*

PT: *That's anger. Fuck you man. Yeah. It's heat and energy.*

TH: *And if that came out at him, what does that anger want to do?*

PT: *Hit him or push him away. "Fuck you, man." You need to make me a man. Show me. Empower me and be a man yourself!*

The fact that he uses the word "fuck" when describing anger, having previously referred to someone as a "mother fucker," suggests some sort of relationship between sex and aggression. These were hints from the unconscious, alerting you to the nature of the conflicts responsible for the patient's struggles.

TH: *So to push him and?*

PT: *Push him and something physical. He stumbles and maybe he falls (laughs). He's in the garden and doesn't know what happened. I am ashamed maybe. I don't know. I'm still a bit angry. I am not through.*

TH: *If it all came out, what else? What else is in your body that wants to come out? Earlier you said kick.*

PT: *I DID say kick.*

TH: *So where do you go for him?*

PT: *On the side, I guess.*

TH: *You guess? When you were first expressing your anger toward your father you kept using the word "fucking," which is an interesting word, suggesting this competitive thing and whether there is room for two dicks in that family* (alluding to the theme of rivalry and competition evident in the example).

PT: (Laughs and nods.) *It's opening something absolutely – when you say, "is there room for two dicks in the family", it's liberating. That's what a father is supposed to do – make his son a man, right?* (The patient is moving toward resolution of the Oedipal conflict – wanting a strong father with whom to identify.)

TH: *And be a solid man himself. And that's what you want – for yourself and your children – so you don't get threatened by conflict.*

PT: *Yeah. Yes. That's why I'm here.*

TH: *So there's a part of you that wants to topple him and even kick him when he's down. And where do you kick him?*

PT: *It's in the crotch – now it's in the crotch. Now he is lying there in the ditch and I'm kicking his crotch (smiling). Oh yeah – whew! It's good. It's like empowering – it's good.* (Shift from anxiety and avoidance to feeling and enjoying the power of his anger.) *This electrifying thing taking over and something in the back saying – "Wow – stop." But still it's coming. It comes in waves and then goes down.*

TH: *So it's really mixed. Part of it feels great, and it's clearly enlivening and strengthening, and it feels good to be on top. It feels good to be strong and to take your place – not to wait for it to be given, but in order to do that you're taking your father down, so there are some feelings about that.*

PT: *Oh yeah, oh yeah.*

TH: *When you see him splayed out and you've been kicking him, what's that feeling?*

As the patient abandoned his defenses and faced his anxiety-provoking and guilt-laden feelings, the de-repression of memories shed light on the development of his conflict and the interpersonal, as well as intrapsychic, manifestations of the same. An unresolved Oedipal conflict, in which he plays the role of the loser, seemed to be in operation. My interventions were designed to test out this hypothesis. His responses will either confirm that hypothesis or prompt a revision.

PT: *Sad. I love him so much (crying and crying). I depended on him for all my life. He has picked me up, picked me up, picked me up again and again (crying). He picks up me and my family. He said, "I'm going to fix this, I'm going to help you". (sobbing). Me and my kids, where would we be without him? It's such mixed emotions. Because he is so detached. You have never met such a detached person.*

Now mixed feelings toward his father were coming to the surface – love and pain, as well as anger. Since the ability to identify with a strong but loving and essentially positive father figure is essential for the resolution of the Oedipal complex, the emergence of these feelings and memories will aid in that process.

TH: *So he does all the right things? Am I understanding this right – he comes in to help or rescue when you are falling down?*

PT: *That's his specialty.*

TH: *His specialty, so what would happen if you are strong and capable and don't need him to come to the rescue?*

PT: *Oooh …*

TH: *Do you want to stay in that needy, one down position, in order to have a relationship with your father?*

PT: *Fuck no. I never thought about it that way.*

TH: *Because now we see that you are actually angry for the ways that he kind of undercut you and kept you dependent. Then there's this wave of sadness and guilt and love, and so what would you want to do in this scenario, when these feelings come up? What shape is he in?*

PT: *He's dumbfounded. I don't know if I got to the part where he really suffered, if you know what I mean.*

TH: *You haven't really faced that – the part of you that would want to inflict some pain.*

PT: *No. Still protecting him. Yeah.*

TH: *What's the price you pay for that?*

PT: *Not being able to be the man of my own life. Holy shit (sigh).*

TH: *What are you really seeing now and what's happening inside?*

PT: *I'm getting angry again. Oh, whew. I don't know how he looks when he suffers and that's a problem. He's never shown it to me.*

TH: *Yeah. So how do you get through to him? He doesn't show you any vulnerability. You are the one who is weak, so he can come to the rescue, right?*

PT: *Even when his wife died* (the woman he married after divorcing the patient's mother) *he said, "I'm going to deal with this in private."!*

TH: *So he won't rely on you or open up to you. No reciprocity and no allowing you to be a strong man he can also lean on. So, this is how you maintained the relationship with your father, as if there was an unconscious contract that you would be weak and stay dependent on him, so he could feel strong. That's his role. And you've been submitting and staying in that one down position. Now you are really angry.*

PT: *Yeah, and surprised. This is not going the way I thought it would. You know, trust toward other guys has been huge for me – like making new friends. I moved to a new city and can't make friends – never, never.*

TH: *When you said, this isn't going the way I thought, you meant the therapy?*

PT: *About my Dad. I didn't realize how pervasive his influence has been. I just thought he was the good guy and Mom was the witch, but of course, I know that he is emotionally unresponsive and that has been irritating me for so long and then the defiant thing, right, "show me something, show me something, come on!". What we are talking about now reminds me of – this connects something in me that I have always identified as anger toward my Mom but now …*

It should be emphasized here that it is **mixed feelings** toward loved ones that must be experienced and integrated for healing to take place. Who can evoke more anger or inflict more searing pain than someone we love? Therapeutic effects rarely result from accessing a single feeling, like anger or grief. Rather, experiencing the inevitably mixed feelings that are evoked toward significant others seems to be required for lasting change. The experience and integration of these feelings lead to resolution of the conflict at hand and allow the patient to see others in a complex, nuanced, and accurate manner. When feelings are defended against, the reality associated with those feelings is distorted. In other words, if you can't face how you feel toward someone and/or about what happened, you will distort what happened to keep those feelings out of consciousness.

This work further strengthened the UTA, providing new material helping us to understand the repeated use of "fuck" and "motherfucker" as he got in touch with anger toward his father. His father seemed to need to keep his son in a one down position in order to feel strong. The patient adopted a passive, submissive, loser stance in response, both to maintain a relationship with his father and to avoid his rage toward him. These unresolved conflicts regarding competition, jealousy, and rivalry often get transmitted from one generation to another. Clearly, in this case, the patient's father had a need to remain in the number one position in the family and to keep his son in a one down, dependent position. The patient had complied with this unconscious demand. Only by accessing his true feelings about this was he able to begin to separate from his father and establish a sense of himself as competent and strong in his own right. Furthermore, this passive submissive stance had been in operation with his wife. He put her wishes before his own, going along both with her desire to have two abortions early in their relationship and agreeing to repeatedly pursue IVF later, in an attempt to replace the lost babies. To behave in this manner, he swallowed all his feelings of anger and turned them back on himself, with depression the result.

An Oedipal Theme Emerges

PT: *Yeah. I spent some vacation time with just my Mom and Dad. I was about 11 and on the verge of puberty. We were going to the mountains to ski, the three of us. I had my own room. The three of us had eaten and downstairs there was a disco and there was music playing and wow, this is so clear* (suggesting the unconscious is wide open). *There was a song by the Gypsy Queens, "Bamboleo, bamboleo." We were sitting at the table after dinner. My Mom kept asking me to dance. I kept saying, "no, no." But now I see today that I'm not as mad as her as I am to my Dad. Of course, I am angry with her for pushing me to do something I don't want to do. I don't want to dance with my Mom – I am 11 years old! With my Mom??? That's kind of perverted and where is my Dad? – he's kind of a shadow.*

TH: *Did she sometimes turn to you because your father wasn't that available? You've been talking about competition. Here is a triangular situation. And again, this use of the word "fuck" when you talk about anger toward your father and mother.*

PT: *Oedipus! Yeah! I have to go to the bathroom.*

TH: *Yeah, and your genitals somehow – there is pressure there, or activation?*

PT: *Yes, yeah. Asserting something.*

TH: *At 11, just getting into puberty. Were you masturbating at that point? Do you remember?*

PT: *Now I'm confused when we talk about that. I am relieved and curious but also a bit like, "Oh, what's going to happen now?" These are things I haven't looked into, so when you say competitive as well … I am getting angry. My butt is getting tight. My sexual relationship with my wife was great for years – fantastic – awesome – until that invitro.* (Patient adds current figure to the mix, allowing for a T-C-P link.)

At this point, the patient's response shows little to no defense in operation. Furthermore, he provided additional information confirming the hypothesis that the conflict in question was sexual and competitive in nature. It is essential for therapists to recognize this as a manifestation of the UTA, a signal to continue to explore the information provided in greater depth.

TH: *Until all that baby stuff.* (Another scenario in which there is a third party vying for the time, attention, and love of the woman in his life).

PT: *Yeah, and all that baby stuff. It's really a* ***graveyard****.*

TH: *That's an interesting word to use.*

PT: *Yeah, graveyard – that's interesting.*

TH: *That's telling. You did actually kill off the first baby, right? You didn't want a third party in the relationship.*

A comment on the use of language is important here. Using emotionally evocative language is intentional, as it serves to intensify the patient's feelings and conflicts, granting deeper access to the unconscious. Speaking to, as well as listening for, the unconscious is of central importance in gaining access to these previously hidden levels of motivation and meaning. In addition, we face, rather than shy away from controversial topics, such as abortion (in this case) and sexual orientation (in the case of the Errant Priest). We must be mindful to listen to, speak to, and understand the patient's conflicts regarding these matters. Imposing our own values, opinions, or political positions is a misuse of our power.

PT: *Wow that hurts. WOOOOO!!! Whew (nodding). That hurts when you say that, but it's true. It's true. It was in a period of my life when I felt strong.*

TH: *And you wanted your girlfriend to yourself. You did not want an intruder, a third party, at that point. Apparently, she agreed, but how did she get pregnant?*

PT: *She said, "Don't worry I'm not going to get pregnant. I've never been pregnant before and I don't use contraception." or something like that. OK. Yeah. We weren't kids you know, we were grownups – 24, 25. (Head in hands) It didn't only happen once. It happened twice.*

TH: *She got pregnant twice?*

PT: *Yeah.*

TH: *So even after she got pregnant, you continued on with no birth control?*

PT: *(shaking his head) Yeah. (sigh) Maybe this is just me being stupid but (sigh), no, this is, uh, I haven't thought about this before – just (motions to push away) – not in this symbolic way.*

TH: *What are you seeing now?*

PT: *It's childish – irresponsible.*

TH: *If you knew what you were doing, but those who do not remember are destined to repeat. You were playing out these unresolved feelings and conflicts that you were completely blind to yet were driving the need to punish yourself.*

PT: *Yeah. Yeah. Not the least is my wife going through all these invitros over and over again. She's been punishing herself too.*

TH: *And trying to undo it – to have two to replace two.*

PT: *Yeah, yeah. Today, yeah. There's probably something sexual about it, because my sexuality has been down for a great while now, so when I feel the adrenaline coming, I guess some testosterone is coming as well.*

TH: *Are you adding things up and putting them together? You're now aware you're also angry at your father. Mixed feelings toward your mother and your wife. How did it link to the graveyard?*

In addition to seeing how he had avoided sexual intimacy as a way of both evading and passively expressing his anger toward his wife, he was able to experience genuine guilt about the previous abortions, instead of simply punishing himself by destroying their sexual connection. He also made a link between that situation in which he did not want an intruder in his relationship to his wife and feelings he had toward his mother in relation to his father. His parents divorced when he was a teenager. His mother moved out of the family home into a cool apartment in the city, where he frequently visited her. He viewed her as hip and interesting in comparison to his stodgy father. He loved being alone with her.

Linking the Present with the Unresolved Past

PT: *I loved it! After a while it got ... she treated me as an adult. We talked about stuff – culture, politics, literature, music. She was bright and interesting and intense, colorful, lively – a bit narcissistic – a great cook.*

TH: *So you really had fun with her. And part of you would be glad to get rid of your father's heavy presence or what?*

PT: *I haven't thought about it, but of course, yeah. That makes sense. Yeah. I haven't thought about that, but I remember for those 3–4 years with my Mom, my Dad was totally in the shadows – even in my life. He would work, sit with a newspaper, eat something, but he was disengaged and just wasn't there.*

TH: *And he was the loser, right? She dumped him and he was a sad sack and that would also be difficult for you to see him be in such a defeated position. In the meantime, you are enjoying having this fun, lively, interesting time with your mother.*

As the patient dropped his defenses and faced his true feelings, memories of what actually transpired emerged. This underscores the point that taking a history prior to the breakthrough can skew the picture and is not advised. In this case, while his parents separated, they didn't divorce for years, leaving everyone in limbo. His feelings shifted as he recalled this material. Initially, he felt a sense of excitement and triumph at having his mother to himself, with his father out of the picture. As the process evolved, he began to feel angry that his parents delayed divorce and did not get on with their lives for many years. Then, the adverse effects of being treated as a partner by his mother were faced.

TH: *You didn't like that he was still in the picture.*

PT: *I didn't like it for him or her. They didn't do each other any good. It wasn't just sexual or competition. I wanted Dad to find someone who could accept him.*

TH: *And he eventually did.*

PT: *Which was fantastic for him, her, and everybody – but then he cared for his cancerous wife instead of me!*

In this last vignette, the patient was able to experience love for his father, suggesting a resolution to the Oedipal conflict. As a result, he was then able to identify with his father and let go of his wish to win his mother's exclusive affection. His father eventually found a loving partner and he was now determined to reconnect with his wife in order to restore their intimacy and closeness. Of course, his unresolved anger toward his wife was also a factor contributing to the distance between them. This underscores the fact that there are often multiple factors contributing to the creation and maintenance of symptoms, a topic we will cover in more depth later in the following chapter.

Furthermore, by allowing himself to experience the guilt over rage toward his father (wanting him dead and out of the picture), and connecting it with guilt over the abortions, he was able to understand how he had created a graveyard with his wife as punishment for getting his wish to have her to himself. The result had been an end to their extremely satisfying sex life, as well as depression and a lack of ambition at work.

The patient left the session feeling tired but alive, clear about the underlying nature of the conflicts responsible for his suffering, and determined to stay connected to his strength and power. Results obtained at a three-year follow-up suggested that his conflicts around anger, competition, and winning had been resolved. He took a stand with his wife that they should adopt their foster child and stop trying to conceive again. Their sexual life became lively and deeply satisfying once again. In addition, he entered a competition for the top spot at work and had no compunction about winning the post as the boss. In fact, he enjoyed being in charge and taking the number one position, both at home and at work. This case illustrated the amount of working through that can happen in a brief period of time, especially when the patient is in a state of crisis.

As the patient was able to face the unresolved past, he was able to achieve mastery over it, freeing himself to shape a new future (Bandura, 2008). No longer viewing himself as a dependent child in need of rescue by his father, but a competent man in his own right, his personal development ensued.

Research suggests that a strong sense of self-efficacy is protective against depression (Maciejewski, Prigerson & Mazure, 2000). Helping patients abandon the defenses of helplessness, passivity, and compliance, which render them vulnerable to repeated episodes of depression, seems to be prophylactic against such recurrence. Since the patient described here had struggled with severe depression in the past, this work was designed to inoculate him against future episodes.

As the transcript suggests, the patient's experience with the therapist was corrective. Her straightforward approach, and communication of confidence in his ability to handle his own feelings, boosted his sense of confidence and stood in stark contrast to the manner in which his father (and previous therapist) had treated him. In the best case scenario, the therapeutic relationship facilitates a process through which impaired or distorted interpersonal relationship schemes are abandoned, reworked, and transformed into more adaptive representations of self and other (Luyten & Blatt, 2011).

Of interest, some research suggests that "Therapeutic progress was associated with increased articulation and differentiation of significant figures, especially mother and therapist ..." (Blatt, Auerbach & Levy, 1996, p. 366). In this case, the patient came into therapy thinking of his mother as a "witch" and his father as his "savior." In alignment with these research findings, the patient increasingly experienced a sense of his mother and therapist as benevolent figures, while seeing his father as more destructive. By the end of this brief but transformational treatment experience, the patient was able to face his very mixed feelings toward both parents (and his wife), resulting in more complex and nuanced perceptions of them. He was able to recover very positive feelings toward his mother and angry feelings toward his father. The latter was particularly important in helping him separate from his father in a healthy manner. In the end, both parents became fully articulated, three-dimensional figures. Not only did he get to the bottom of his depression and anxiety, but was able to rework his own sense of self. No longer sentenced to living life in a cage, he had freed himself to become active, connected, and successful both at work and at home.

Creating an Intrapsychic Crisis in Patients with Chronic Difficulties

The Errant Priest

While the patient just described entered treatment in a state of crisis, this middle-aged priest had long-standing difficulties and was mired in a chronic pattern of defensiveness. He requested a consultation when a previous 60-session treatment resulted in a worsening of his presenting complaints. I agreed to an initial session over Zoom, as he lived a great distance from my office and was unable to travel for a trial therapy. The intention was to get some sense of him and his difficulties so that I could make a good referral. Having had one negative experience with therapy, I had hoped to find a good match for him. This was my first attempt at using Zoom – something that would become routine when Covid restrictions prevented us from meeting in person.

FIRST SESSION

The patient started by reporting a compulsion to watch homosexual pornography, which was highly disturbing to him. We began with an inquiry into the precipitants, in an effort to uncover the cause or causes of this behavior.

TH: *You say this all started three years ago. What was happening at that time?*

PT: *They moved me from where I had been working to another state. It is very rural and small. I was sent to live in a community with all these old Priests. It was very lonely for me. I finally told my Superior that I had to go and couldn't stand it there. He said he understood but couldn't find another post for me, so I had to make it work.*

TH: *That sounds terrible. You must have had a lot of feelings toward your superiors.*

PT: *Well, that's just the way it is, so I figured I'd have to make it work, but then I found out that all these Priests were living a double life* (having homosexual relations, even with each other).

TH: *So how do you feel about being placed there?*

PT: *I was sad. I was frustrated, I suppose. Then, strangely enough, I started to act like them – having a double life.*

TH: *That's what we need to understand, isn't it?*

PT: *Yes. But it's very strange. When I was young, I fell in love with girls. I didn't see myself as homosexual. This was all really confusing and upsetting, so that's why I started to see the other therapist.*

TH: *What did you get out of that treatment? Was it helpful?*

PT: *Yes, but it got worse. After the therapy – or actually during the therapy – I started to go to chat rooms and even hook up with guys. It was awful.*

TH: *What happened?*

PT: *I didn't want to do it, but I would do it. I would go meet someone and they would start something, and I wouldn't say no. It's not enjoyable for me. It's painful. I didn't want to do it, but I would submit to it.*

TH: *It sounds really painful – almost punitive. The question is, for what?*

PT: *I don't know. It was just so painful living as I was. I was so lonely.*

TH: *So, on the one hand, in order to avoid all the feelings about being in such a place, with men who are living double lives, you adopt a kind of "if you can't beat 'em, join 'em" attitude. It sounds like it was so intolerable to be so alone, that you took desperate measures to connect.*

The first obvious precipitant to this symptomatic behavior was a painful feeling of loneliness resulting from the loss of everyone he knew and loved. Of interest, when placed in a rectory with older priests, most of whom were leading double lives and conducting homosexual relationships, he followed suit. Was this just a way to ward off feelings of isolation and to become a part of something? Surely it couldn't be that simple. The patient provided a clue.

PT: *Yes, I was left alone by my Superior and left by my father.*

TH: *Your father?*

PT: *He left when I was a young baby and was never in my life. It turns out he was an alcoholic.*

TH: *So there is pain and a longing for closeness, but there must also be …*

PT: *And you know what else happened – the reason I was moved – is because the Pastor I was working with, who was my best friend, died suddenly in an accident.*

TH: *What happened?*

PT: *He fell down the stairs and broke his neck.*

TH: *How did that affect you?*

PT: *I started acting out after his death. Suddenly I was fascinated by men's bodies. I am still acting out. I don't want to, but I do it. I only feel pain. It's almost as if I am destroying myself because living is too painful. I am profoundly sad.*

TH: *How do you feel that pain and sadness?*

PT: *It's a profound sadness in my heart and my chest.*

TH: *So, pain and grief over this huge and sudden loss is one thing, but needing to destroy yourself, as you are doing now, is something else. This is what we need to understand. You lost your best friend and then lost everything – your parish and home. They sent you off to the middle of nowhere to live with these old men who are living a double life. I wonder if you are just sad.*

PT: *No – I am angry – I am really angry! How could God take away such a good man? I am really angry at God. He was a good man and didn't break the rules – but he dies! I am so mad.*

TH: *How do you experience that anger?*

PT: *I am angry and I am just going to be disobedient!*

TH: *So how do you do that?*

PT: *Oh my God, by doing the worst thing imaginable. It's a sin.*

TH: *So you act out your anger by being the bad boy. Then who suffers?*

PT: *I do. But if God can be cruel, I can be too. Yes. Yes. At times, I think I'm just going to quit this world. The only way to be free is to die.*

TH: *That would be the ultimate punishment – to take yourself out.*

PT: *Suddenly I got the image of me with a gun and a vision of killing other people and killing the priests I am living with.*

Both the conscious and unconscious alliances were very strong at this point, revealing information that helped us understand the origin of his difficulties. His compulsive behavior was alien and dystonic, causing him enormous pain and anguish, as well as confusion. We were beginning to understand and make sense of behavior that baffled him previously.

TH: *So you do it to yourself instead. It's a way of protecting others from your violent rage and a way to punish yourself all at the same time.*

PT: *This is amazing. It's all making so much sense. I would rather destroy myself than other people. I feel a tremendous relief right now.*

TH: *It seems we've gotten to at least some of the origins of these highly distressing symptoms.*

PT: *Yes, it's starting to make sense. I just couldn't understand it and we never got to any of this in my previous therapy* (with a female therapist).

TH: *You must have lots of feelings toward her.*

PT: *She was very strict and demanding – telling me I had to leave the priesthood and should take up a homosexual lifestyle. I would go along with her in the sessions, but then act out during the week.*

TH: *It sounds like you have a tendency to be compliant – like doing what the other priests in your house are doing – but then defiant as well – acting out in anger against God and your former therapist.*

PT: *That is true, I am afraid. It's like I never grew up. I went to the seminary right out of high school. I want to be my own man.*

TH: *So, in addition to sorting out all your feelings about the events of the last three years, instead of acting them out in such a destructive manner you want to stand on your own two feet and be a man of your own making.*

PT: *Yes, that would be great.*

In addition to gaining agreement about the problems to be addressed, we must obtain consensus about goals and the tasks required to attain rather than sabotage them.

TH: *Well, I think we've gotten a sense of some of the factors that are responsible for this crisis. Now that I have a sense of you and what kind of help you need, I can make a referral to someone in your area.*

PT: *No! No! Can't we continue? I got more out of this one hour than sixty sessions with that other therapist. I think we are getting to the heart of the matter. Would it be possible?*

TH: *Well, I haven't done a treatment online before, but we could give it a try and keep assessing if it's useful to you. How does that sound?*

PT: *Fantastic.*

TH: *You really spoke up for what you wanted and needed, rather than submitting to my suggestion for a referral. That seems new.*

PT: *Yes, and it feels great.*

Much was revealed during this first session, and a great deal was accomplished, including a corrective experience at the end of the session when I responded positively to his request, instead of rejecting it out of hand (as had his Superior in the Order). It seemed as if the original symptom of compulsive pornography use had multiple sources. This behavior proved a powerful distraction and means of avoiding pain and grief about the loss of his beloved friend, his home, and his religious community. Additionally, the sudden loss of his friend and mentor who was literally a "father" to him (this is how priests are addressed) seemed to revive long dormant feelings from his own father who abandoned him at an early age. When elaborating upon his "fascination with male bodies," he reported being particularly interested in the man's face, chest, and arms, realizing that his deepest longing was to be held securely in the arms of a strong man while gazing into his eyes. This material reinforced the notion that a longing for closeness with an absent father was a significant factor involved in the creation of his symptoms.

In addition, we were also able to identify the ways in which watching homosexual pornography served as a disguised expression of anger toward the Superiors who sent him off to an isolated parish and the God who took his friend away. At the same time, indulging in behavior that caused him great anguish and was at odds with his own values, functioned as a means of punishing himself for that anger. He experienced anger as dangerous and revealed a fear that he might act out violently if he allowed himself to feel this rage.

Finally, when sent away to an isolated location with priests who were all acting out, he avoided his pain and rage via a process of identification – becoming like them. Of note, the patient could identify his emotions and the impulses associated with them but tended to avoid the actual, visceral experience of these feelings. In this case, acting out was a compromise between the desire to express his anxiety-provoking and guilt-laden feelings, while defending against the internal experience of them. Rather than face his inner drama, he created drama in his external life. Helping him to experience, tolerate, and integrate his strong mixed feelings toward others was a central therapeutic task and goal.

While the pornography use started after the loss of his friend and reassignment to a rural outpost, having actual sexual contacts with men did not begin until he entered his first psychotherapy. Consequently, feelings toward his previous therapist needed to be explored in subsequent sessions.

Summary

Vignettes from two initial sessions were used to illustrate the ways in which "working through" can take place from the start of treatment. Neither insight nor emotional catharsis alone is sufficient to create deep and lasting change. Rather, a complex series of interventions and therapeutic processes are required. These include (1) turning patients on destructive defenses, (2) facilitating the visceral experience of complex mixed feelings toward others, and (3) linking current symptoms and troubling behavior to unresolved conflicts from the past.

In the first case, the patient was in crisis and highly motivated to face what he had been avoiding. Four hours were sufficient to resolve his conflicts and reignite stalled development. In the second case, a one-hour consultation mobilized the conscious and unconscious alliances in a patient who had only gotten worse in a previous therapy and set the stage for a longer, but ultimately successful, treatment. In each case, deep insight followed the breakdown of defenses and breakthrough of previously avoided feelings, a process vital to achieving deep and lasting change.

Chapter 3

Complexity and Multiple Causation

Human beings are complicated, and life is messy. So too is psychotherapy and the process of change. All too often, we seek simple solutions to complex problems, reducing our understanding of psychological disturbances to a single factor such as dysfunctional beliefs or guilt over rage toward loved ones. In this chapter, the idea that human suffering is a manifestation of significant complexity, with many contributing factors and layers of meaning, will be elucidated. The psychoanalytic concepts of multiple causation and overdetermination will aid in our understanding of symptoms and pathological behaviors. Furthermore, the necessity for assessing and working through these layers of motivation and meaning in order to achieve deep and lasting change will be emphasized. This often requires multiple types and levels of intervention. Finally, the process of identifying and working through multiple factors will be illustrated with detailed case examples.

Multiple Causation and Overdetermination

In *The Interpretation of Dreams* (1900), Freud suggested that, contrary to popular belief, dreams were not mere nonsense but had significant and often complex meanings. In addition, he posited that certain images were overdetermined. In other words, a single image or theme was viewed as being determined by multiple factors, any one of which would be sufficient to account for the effect.

Similarly, symptoms and character traits can be, and often are, "overdetermined" by multiple factors. For example, a conversion symptom such as the paralysis of the right arm might be caused by identification with a crippled mother, *and represent* guilt over the desire to take a knife and plunge it into the heart of said mother. Furthermore, the patient, who might have been enlisted into a care-taking role with her mother, could, by becoming incapacitated, find a way out of this role *and* manage to get some attention for herself. While any of these four factors alone could determine the formation of such a symptom, in many cases, several motives are involved; all of which must be uncovered in order for healing to take place. Once all the

DOI: 10.4324/9781003197669-3

contributing factors have been identified, the patient's willingness to explore them and, ultimately, give them up in favor of health and healing will be required for lasting change.

Cyclical psychodynamics (Butler & Binder, 1987; Wachtel, 1997, 2014) is a comprehensive model of psychopathology that incorporates both intrapsychic (triangle of conflict) and interpersonal (triangle of person) factors, in an attempt to understand both the original cause of symptoms and the mechanisms that perpetuate them. This integrated model is "an attempt at improved specification of the principles and procedures implicit in the creation of a comprehensive psychodynamic formulation" (Butler & Binder, 1987, p. 218). Unlike traditional psychoanalytic models that regard current difficulties as a direct manifestation of early trauma, cyclical psychodynamics suggests that the patient's current problems are the inevitable result of vicious cycles of psychological reactivity and behavior that are "self-defeating, self-perpetuating, relatively inflexible and maladaptive" (Strupp & Binder, 1984, p. 217). According to Wachtel (1993), emotional conflicts, unconscious motivation, interpersonal relationships, and behavior interact in a mutual and reciprocal fashion. In other words, the patient's current difficulties are understood as a manifestation of "a salient pattern of interpersonal roles in which patients unconsciously cast themselves and others" (Butler and Binder, 1987, p. 219) in such a way that his worst fears are repeatedly confirmed.

According to this theory, while symptoms may originally be caused by emotional conflicts in the past, they are perpetuated by rigid patterns of (defensive) interaction which perpetuate the patient's suffering. Given this, simply understanding the original source of the conflict often proves incomplete. In addition, the patient must come to see the ways in which he habitually replays these old, outmoded, and destructive patterns in his current life, pulling for the very responses he dreads (as was demonstrated in the case of "The Man in the Cage," Chapter 1). As Edna St Vincent Millay observed, "It's not true that life is one damn thing after the other. It is the same damn thing, over and over" (Macdougall, 1952).

Understanding these dysfunctional patterns of reactivity and behavior is essential, but frequently inadequate for the promotion of lasting change. Patients often enact their conflicts with the therapist by unconsciously inviting him to repeat and reinforce these destructive patterns of interaction with them (Weiss, 1993). Weiss (1993) took an empirical approach to the study of psychotherapy and psychoanalysis, concluding that the therapist's primary task involved helping patients disprove the pathological beliefs that prohibited them from pursuing desired but forbidden goals. This notion is similar to what Balint (1968) called a "counteroffer" or what Alexander and French (1946) referred to as a "corrective emotional experience."

By contradicting the patient's expectations and providing a new experience, several tasks are accomplished.

Freud hypothesized that we feel in the contrast, not in the state of things. When we respond in a new and unexpected way to the patient's bid for a replay of a pathological pattern, it often evokes strong feelings. Since the creation of a highly charged emotional atmosphere is associated with positive outcomes, evoking such feelings within the therapeutic relationship is of vital importance. Furthermore, the activation of these feelings often provides an opening into the unconscious, triggering memories, dreams, and associations that shed light on the origin of the patient's conflicts. Often, pathological beliefs associated with de-repressed affect can be reevaluated in the light of this new and contradictory experience (Ecker et al., 2012). So, just as multiple factors are responsible for the creation and maintenance of symptoms and character traits, multiple therapeutic factors are responsible for altering them.

Let's consider the example of a depressed young man of 30. As a child, he was consistently punished for aggressive behavior and learned to suppress his angry impulses, covering them up with the defenses of compliance and passivity. These defenses reduced anxiety and were actively reinforced by his parents. A mutual and reciprocal interplay of interpersonal and intrapsychic factors would contribute to the creation and maintenance of this man's depression, since passivity had become over-generalized and calcified into a habitual way of being. By suppressing all of his own anger and desires, and subsequently having developed no sense of agency or confidence, he would be set up for recurring depression. Such was the case with "The Man in a Cage", detailed in the previous chapter.

Human beings are meaning-making machines. We create narratives and tell stories in an attempt to understand ourselves, others, and the world around us. These stories often become self-fulfilling prophecies. If this hypothetical young man told himself that he is not as good as others and must maintain a one-down position, it will likely become a self-fulfilling prophecy. Furthermore, behaving in a passive and compliant fashion invites others to assume a more dominant role in the interaction. This only confirms his sense of inadequacy and fuels his depression, perpetuating the cycle.

It is up to the therapist to interrupt, rather than reinforce, this type of dysfunctional pattern. While resisting the pull to take over and become too dominant, the therapist might say something like, "I simply don't buy this façade of passivity. What is it that you really want?" or "Do you see how, by remaining passive and waiting for me to start the session, you invite me to take over and leave you in the lurch? Is that what you want to play out here or should we do it differently?"

To reiterate, it is of the utmost importance to remember that, just as there are multiple factors involved in the causation and perpetuation of suffering, there are multiple factors involved in removing it and replacing it with healthy alternatives. Both the intrapsychic and interpersonal aspects of functioning must be addressed in order to create sustained change. In the therapeutic process, this typically involves the facilitation of previously avoided and anxiety-laden feelings, the development of insight into the links between current and past behaviors, a corrective emotional experience with a therapist, and the attainment of new perspectives and possibilities.

Cultural, genetic, and temperamental factors must also be taken into consideration. In some cases, symptoms have become functionally autonomous and have taken on a life of their own, no longer simply triggered by emotional conflicts. In such cases, behavioral approaches might also have a role to play in the treatment plan. This is especially true in cases of addiction, for example. This interplay of therapeutic factors is often required to produce profound and permanent alteration in the psychological life of our patients.

Ultimately, it is the response to intervention that lets us know when we have hit "pay dirt" or must continue our search for the relevant factors responsible for the patient's difficulties. We gather data on the nature, history, and severity of the symptoms; form a hypothesis; and then test it out with our interventions. The patient's response to our intervention, especially the lifting of the target symptom, gives us the most reliable and timely data on our effectiveness.

The Man Who Couldn't Stop Shaking

This 50-year-old married father of four came to see the therapist after being released from a day treatment program. While functioning well most of his adult life as an executive with a national company, he had been unrelentingly depressed for the previous two years (since the death of his mother) and was on disability when he arrived for outpatient treatment. Of note, this depression included a nearly constant inner dialog about his worthlessness, along with a demand that he should kill himself.

His first depression, which included psychotic features, occurred during his first year of college. Depression had plagued him throughout his life but had not been as incapacitating as this most recent episode, which had required two hospitalizations, a day treatment program, and various forms of outpatient psychotherapy and medication. Since he had not responded to any of these previous treatments in any significant way, he was referred to me, in the hopes that Intensive Short-Term Dynamic Psychotherapy (ISTDP) might be effective.

In fact, he responded extremely well to our first three sessions. In each case, as defenses of passivity, helplessness, internalization, and rationalization were abandoned, and his true feelings of pain, rage, and guilt were experienced, he felt an immediate lifting of the depression – something he had never experienced previously. This greatly increased his hope and motivation. In addition to symptom reduction, he demonstrated character change by beginning to speak up and assert himself at home with his wife and children. Unfortunately, they did not respond positively and put pressure on him to resume his subservient role in the family. This clearly provoked a crisis within him, as he entered the fourth session visibly shaking in an uncontrolled manner.

Session #4

PT: *I am experiencing some anxiety.*
TH: *I see that. What are you noticing with the anxiety inside?*
PT: *This* (referring to his body shaking).
TH: *That's almost a way to get discharge or get rid of it – how do you feel the anxiety inside?*
PT: *I don't know what you mean.*
TH: *Other than the shaking, anything else you notice?*
PT: *No.*
TH: *So you say it started a few days ago? What was going on?*

To ascertain the nature of the conflict responsible for the symptom, specific information about triggering situations is essential to obtain.

PT: *It happened the other day, then it wasn't happening.*
TH: *So it's been waxing and waning?*
PT: *Yeah, oftentimes – Jesus, I'm sorry.*
TH: *No need to apologize. There is a lot of feeling under there. Let's see what's triggering it – there is a lot of feeling.*
PT: *It has a lot to do with – oftentimes, it's about work, or that I'm not working, and thinking about going back to work. It also has something to do with coming here or going to a Dr's appointment.*
TH: *It stirs up lots of feelings.*
PT: *But I don't understand what they are.*
TH: *So let's see if we can find out what feelings are there underneath all this tension and anxiety that is causing this kind of distress. What kinds of feelings do you have about being here today?*
PT: *I think it has to do with facing my situation. Facing that I am not right yet.*
TH: *To face what is inside – facing all the feelings you have been avoiding. What kind of feelings do you have here toward me?*
PT: *There you go again. It's not about you, it's about me.*
TH: *But it only happens at certain times, like when you are here with me or with your primary physician. It's just a trigger. Coming here is a trigger. On the one hand, you are here to get better and want relief, but in order to get there, you have to go through some difficult things and face some difficult feelings. Right?*
PT: *(sigh) That makes logical sense but it's just not resonating.*

Even though there was evidence suggesting that the patient was experiencing anger toward me that was triggering his anxiety at the moment, he did not seem to agree. Since he had a history of compliance with others, the fact that he was able to say, "No, it's not resonating with me," was something I wanted to support. Instead of insisting on my point of view, I demonstrated interest in his.

TH: *What's your hypothesis?*
PT: *I don't have one. When I'm like this I have difficulty understanding it. I am reasonably intelligent, but I feel like a moron.*
TH: *Then there is self-attack on top of it. Obviously, you are suffering.*
PT: *And I have been* (head in hands) ... *This past week I've been really, um, the stuff about "you should kill yourself" has been really bad.*

Of note, these suicidal thoughts had completely disappeared after our first session. It was not yet clear what had precipitated their return. Rather than assuming I already knew the cause of his distress, or persisting in making a case for my theory, I encouraged his engagement and remained open and flexible in response. More inquiry would be required to discover the underlying cause of his symptoms.

TH: *Really bad. OK, so could we agree that all this – the self-attack, telling yourself you should die, being wracked with anxiety and shaking – is pretty tortuous and punitive, wouldn't you say?* (This was an attempt to get agreement about the problem and the task, so we are working collaboratively and not at cross purposes.)
PT: *Yeah.*
TH: *So the question is, what are you punishing yourself for? Isn't that what we want to discover – why would you need to treat yourself this way?*
PT: *(heavy breathing) OK – we can agree (laughing), sure (throws up his hands).*
TH: *I really don't want you to just go along with me. I am trying to understand your experience. It sounds pretty torturous to me.*

It is of the utmost importance that the therapist refuse to repeat the pattern of taking a dominant role, while demanding patient compliance. Rather, working to create agreement about the tasks required and goals to be achieved is required to solidify a truly collaborative alliance. Since the patient's helplessness and despair were quite syntonic, challenging them at that time would be contraindicated. More work was required to gain agreement on the therapeutic tasks ahead.

PT: *The thing about it is, yes, but it's become such a norm for me (crying and shaking). Jesus, it's such a back slide (starts to weep). I'm just so sad, I am so sad.*

Patience paid off. Since the therapist did not engage in an interpersonal battle of wills, but remained focused on understanding the patient's suffering, the patient was left to struggle with his own inner conflict. His defenses broke down and deep feelings of grief broke through.

TH: *Just let that through – so much pain and grief for all you've lost.*
PT: *(Weeping for several minutes) I don't even know what this is.*
TH: *There is a tremendous amount of emotional pain inside and you just can't contain it anymore.*
PT: *(Sobbing) I don't even know what it is. It would be one thing if I could just say, "This happened and I am sad." I don't understand it. I am just this way. I am just this way.*

The patient was not yet able to understand his own emotional response and was overgeneralizing, using his experience in order to reinforce his view of himself as inherently damaged in some sort of permanent way. He thought his depression represented who he was, rather than being the result of what he was doing – defending against his painful and anxiety-provoking feelings. Helping him to distinguish between who he is as a human being and what he does was of vital importance. This underscores the fact that it is not enough to help patients feel their feelings but to develop a deep understanding of what these feelings reveal, so that we can integrate and consolidate this information into a coherent sense of self.

TH: *Well, what does come to mind when you let yourself feel this pain and sorrow?*
PT: *I just feel shit. I just feel. Ah, I'm just trying so hard not to feel this.*
TH: *But isn't that …*
PT: *Of course, of course. That's easy to say afterward, but it's just so hard.*
TH: *But you're calmer after, do you notice?*
PT: *Again, it would be one thing if I could pinpoint a certain thing.*

In this vignette, the patient evidenced an awareness of the ways in which his avoidance of pain had created and perpetuated suffering. The precipitous drop in anxiety and shaking, as he allowed himself to feel emotional pain, was striking and needed to be emphasized. Furthermore, he would need help to understand his emotional states, as well as regulating them. While the patient was not yet able to understand the grief he was feeling, the therapist had obtained information in previous sessions that could help them make sense of it. She decided to share this understanding with the patient, in order to keep the process moving forward.

TH: *But there are many things, right? You have lost a lot – not only people, but a sense of direction, meaning, and purpose. Your father died when you were quite young, you don't like your work, and your marriage is very difficult. There is a lot of pain and grief there, isn't there?*

PT: *Yes! Yeah! Jesus, I didn't expect this* (patient sighs and visibly relaxes, with no shaking of any kind visible).

TH: *It's striking how much calmer you are now. It's trying to keep it all tightly bound and under wraps, telling yourself you have no reason to feel this – it's created a tremendous conflict.*

PT: *I absolutely agree with what you're saying. The way I would describe it is, how do I say this, it's almost as though I can only recognize it after the fact – what I have been repressing. I've been that way for so long. I am left-handed. It would be like I would never think to write with my right hand.*

TH: *You mean you have been so detached from your feelings for so long, to feel seems foreign.*

Here it was emphasized that he had been DOING something that exacerbated his suffering, in contrast to the notion that he was "just this way." His ability to reflect and make sense of his experience was far greater *after* the breakthrough of feeling, than during the initial encounter, when he was expending energy to contain and repress his true feelings. His ability to engage in the therapeutic task had been hindered by these defensive efforts but were freed up once defenses were relinquished.

PT: *Yeah. And, I mean, that sucks. Whew! The realization that it has caused me so much harm.*

TH: *The very thing you did to …*

PT: *To survive, yeah.*

TH: *Like when your father died, and your mother got so depressed. You shut it all down. All the energy it takes to keep it contained and then this shaking and eruption.*

PT: *I did not expect this today. Holy crap! (sigh) I feel so much better! (laughs with relief)*

The patient was not only freeing himself to feel his emotions but was starting to understand himself in a new and ultimately liberating way. At first, he was baffled and couldn't make sense of his symptoms. Then he concluded, "This is just the way I am." With help, he was beginning to see that he had developed ways of coping during childhood that had persisted over time. Furthermore, he was able to understand that the very strategies he had used to survive in childhood had caused pain and suffering in his adult life. This recognition was painful but hopeful at the same time. He experienced massive relief. Now the insights and connections between past and present, defenses and symptoms, needed to be expanded and reinforced.

TH: *So this is the cycle – shove, shove, shove, with all the feelings building up until you are ready to blow, often in anger. Then you feel terrible and start suppressing again.*
PT: *Right.*
TH: *So we want to try and create this connection between you and you so you can develop an intimate relationship with you and know what you are feeling on an ongoing basis instead of this all or nothing.*
PT: *Yeah – all or nothing – you really said something there. I have to teach myself to check in. That's really going to be hard. How can I do that?*
TH: *Let's see if you can stay connected. How are you aware of feeling right now?*
PT: *I feel calm. My head is saying, "You have to crack this puzzle." I go to my head and that's really not the thing to do.*

The preceding statement suggested that the patient was increasingly able to catch his own defenses as they arose. He could see that going to his head and demanding performance – a strategy that no longer served him. Actively supporting and reinforcing such healthy shifts is vital to consolidating change.

TH: *How great that you noticed that – that you habitually detach and go to your head to figure it out.*
PT: *Exactly (smiling and delighted). Wow – instead of just being. I've got to nurture myself.*
TH: *And others.*
PT: *I have rejected the emotional connection with others, and rarely connect with myself.* (Revealing enhanced insight and a lack of defensiveness.)
TH: *How can you stay connected in an ongoing way?*
PT: *Can you give me the answer?* (Testing out whether I will come in as the expert, reinforcing his view of himself as inadequate.)
TH: *Let's do it, instead of just talking about it. How do you notice feeling in this moment?*
PT: *I am trying to focus on it. I am starting to feel a tingling. There was tension that has been released. I am also feeling a little silly for having this – but I caught it.*
TH: *That's an angry, vicious voice.*
PT: *It really is.*
TH: *It's being turned on you. It begs the question, who is that anger really toward? Who are you really angry with?*
PT: *That voice is always there with me.*
TH: *You weren't born with it. Do you remember when it came online?*

PT: *At times, I think it's my mother. It's almost as though it has the same essence – not her actual voice in my head. The sense of shame. I always felt this weird sense of shame.*

TH: *About what?*

PT: *I don't know. She had this way of ... as I was about to tell you and the voice says, "What a cliché – you are in a Psychologist's office talking about your mother."*

TH: *So it's really dismissive.*

PT: *Yes, yes! It really is. Jesus.* (Separating himself from the defense of self-attack and feeling the cost.)

TH: *You're beginning to catch it and realize it's a running commentary.*

The fact that the patient was able to recognize his own defenses, and their negative consequences, was very good news. Furthermore, he was starting to turn on them without being excessively harsh or critical of himself in the process. New memories shedding light on the development of these conflicts emerged.

PT: *She would do this thing, if you were doing something wrong, she would give you this look. My sibs and I talked about it. I felt myself shrinking, like I did something wrong. That was pervasive. I always felt I was doing something wrong. I could blame her, but it doesn't help.*

TH: *It's not about blaming her but facing what happened and your feelings about it. You remember the look. Was it contemptuous?*

PT: *Contemptuous – that's it! Wow. Contemptuous. Oh man. There was this, "how dare you," to it.*

TH: *What would trigger that?*

PT: *It wouldn't matter. I remember painting a watercolor and simply didn't clean up fast enough, or I ate with my fingers as a 5-year-old. She wasn't an awful woman, but when I was little, I felt ashamed all the time. What's important is that I've internalized it. It has that essence – that message.*

TH: *You said that your mother was very depressed. Did you say she needed ECT?*

I inquired about his history in order to understand all the factors involved in his having shut down at such a young age. While I knew there was a history of depression in the family (both his mother and sister required ECT), I did not know the details. Given the opening in this session, we explored this further.

PT: *She even needed it before I was born. My sister died at the age of 4. After my Mom died, my aunt died. We found photos of my sister that were too painful for my mother to have around so my Aunt had them. All these photos of my mother as a young woman with a child that we had never seen.*

A couple, in particular, were taken just before my sister died. My mother was young, slender, radiant, and happy. My God, I thought, who is this happy woman? I never saw that woman. I never saw that. It was stunning. When you think about how devastating. After she died, after the funeral, a cousin described the day my sister died from pneumonia. They described the screaming from my mother – like a wild animal. Everything changed. My Mom stopped eating and was catatonic, so they did ECT. Years later, in high school, we saw a program about ECT and how brutal it was in those days. "That's what happened to me," she said. That was almost a moment of acceptance.

TH: *And a certain closeness.*

PT: *In a big way. There is a lot of anger and frustration at my Mom but knowing what she went through ... She went through so much and was as strong as anyone I know. She was also weak and fragile.* (Increased ability to tolerate ambivalence.)

TH: *She had a lot to deal with – the death of a child and her husband.*

PT: *How did we get here?* (Alerting us to the need to connect, understand, and create coherence.)

TH: *We're trying to understand the origin of this harsh, critical voice, and you remember the look from your mother and how you would wilt. It's not about vilifying her but understanding the impact on you as a child – what happened AND what you made that mean.*

PT: *Exactly.*

TH: *You thought it was you – you were wrong – but it had nothing to do with you. It had to do with her state of mind.*

PT: *I've known this on some level, but the emotional impact is new.* (It is emotional insight, not cognitive insight, that is most strongly associated with lasting change.)

TH: *The intellectual understanding isn't enough, but to come to terms with all the feelings as well. There was a lot of feeling as you told me about that. How do you feel now?*

PT: *It's strange. It's a sense of loss – I mourn for her and for me, that I never got that happy mother.* (A sense of understanding and compassion is replacing his harsh and critical inner voice.)

TH: *So that deep pain you had coming in – you didn't know what it was about – it was a deep loss from the start – the loss of a mother who was unburdened.*

PT: *A heavy burden from the day I was born. That's what it was. Some metaphor about a heavy cloak. I had a heavy cloak upon me from the beginning.*

TH: *How could you ever make up for that? You were destined to fail. You could never make her happy. It gets replicated now with your wife – the sense you can never make her happy.* (Unfortunately, his wife confirmed rather than refuted this notion, complaining about him and attributing her unhappiness and that of the children solely to his actions.)

PT: *As I am sitting here and experiencing silence in a way I rarely do. It's quiet and peaceful.*

TH: *When did you notice that?*

PT: *After you said what you just said. All the rushing thoughts are gone.*

While we obviously want the patient's symptoms to disappear, that alone is not enough to ensure ongoing progress. A deep understanding of what caused the symptoms, as well as what was required to remove them, seems to be necessary for lasting change to take place. The preceding transcript suggested that defenses and symptoms were being replaced with healthy alternatives. In particular, his harsh and critical inner voice was being replaced with understanding and compassion, both for himself and his mother.

TH: *What do you make of that?*

PT: *It's another whirlwind session. It's about sitting with it all. Why does it have to get to "you should kill yourself only one set of? Why should I give that voice power?"*

TH: *How do you make sense of it?*

PT: *It's contemptuous. Her – whatever message I was taking in had nothing to do with me. I've understood that intellectually. It's like there are two of me.*

TH: *One is an occupier – intrusive – not who you really are. You want to be free of that. You weren't put on the planet to make your mother happy or make up for your sister's death. You must find your own reason for living.*

PT: *I don't know that I ever felt what you are describing, but on some level that is what it was. The feeling was, "I'm not enough." That's what it was. I described to you last time, how I thought I could be me once she was gone. I actually believed that for years - that when she was gone, I would be free. This is all coming together. I wish it had come together 20 years ago, but here we are (pause). There's the silence again, and there is no internal dialog or criticism.*

TH: *How is it just to be quiet and peaceful?*

PT: *It's quiet. Now I started to see, "figure out what you're going to do?" But it's Ok, I can just sit with this.*

TH: *And when you get to the point of asking yourself what you WANT to do, not should do …*

PT: *What a great question – what I want to do! What do I FEEL like? I have to place importance on that because I have ignored it for so long.*

TH: *It also sounds like you've associated anxiety and guilt with your own feelings and wishes, so you've been at war. To be free of that and to discover who you are and what you really want.*

PT: *This is great, sitting here. What I have to do is keep it going in my own life.*

Therapy with patients who suffer from chronic depression and character disorders is extremely challenging, due to the entrenched patterns of self-defeating behavior that are often repeated in relation to the therapist (Bourke & Grenyer, 2010; Hollon, Thase & Markowitz, 2002). Rather than viewing such patterns as an obstacle to treatment, attention to the transference pattern of behavior affords patient and therapist the ability to deal with the conflict directly, in the here and now. Such immediacy is associated with positive outcome (Clemence et al., 2011; Kasper, Hill & Kilvkighan, 2008).

Character defenses such as compliance, subservience, hopelessness, and helplessness must be repeatedly addressed and ultimately removed, lest the patterns that rendered him susceptible to a recurrence of depression remain intact. Masterson (1990) emphasized that such character disorders constitute a false self, constructed from the child's desire to please the mother. In this case, pleasing his mother was an impossible task. The patient could never replace his dead sister (or his father). His failure to make his mother happy and lift her depression led to a profound sense of worthlessness within him.

His own depression clearly had many sources, including self-directed anger, punishment for guilt over his angry, destructive wishes, pathological mourning, and a possible introjection of his mother's death wish toward him. Could it be that she wanted to get rid of this boy, who could not possibly replace her dead daughter? Derek Miller (personal communication, 1980) suggested, in contrast to the more popular notion of suicide as a murderous wish turned toward the self, he believed that "no one kills himself who someone else didn't want dead." The patient was so compliant – so desperate to please – we might wonder if his wish to "off" himself was a manifestation of just such a dynamic. Might it have also been an enactment of his wife's wish? She regarded him as a burden, yet undercut all his efforts at self-expression and assertion.

Many factors had conspired in the development of both passivity and depression in this man. There was pathological mourning, both for his father and the happy mother he never knew; a tendency to protect others and turn his anger inward; guilt over this anger, which demanded punishment; identification with a depressed mother; and assuming responsibility for her depression. All these elements needed to become conscious so that they could be reevaluated and revised anew. Many factors were required to help him resolve these conflicts and free himself from suffering, including abandoning defenses that hurt him, distinguishing who he was from what he did to defend himself, facing and integrating mixed feelings toward others, and developing understanding and compassion for himself and others.

The Immigrant

This 40-year-old professional man came from a significant distance for a three-day block therapy. We met two hours each day, for a total of six therapy hours. I had obtained no information prior to our meeting so that I could assess him in real time.

Hour I

TH: *Start with why you're here. What brings you?*

PT: *I have impotence – not having any sexual pleasure. I have been married two times. I have been married twice. This is my second marriage. I am married for the second time for two years. We have been together for one year now and it's not good. I cannot get an erection.*

TH: *At all?*

PT: *I get it but then can't keep it.*

TH: *Ever?*

PT: *No, that's right.*

TH: *So, it's been from the start. And what about your 1st marriage?*

PT: *It was not good. I am 42 years old and had sex maybe 10 times.*

TH: *Why was that?*

PT: *Health issues. From childhood I have been suffering from depression. During my first marriage it was a major issue. I was suicidal. I was contemplating suicide every hour of the day. My first memory of me being suicidal was at 5 years old. That time – 2 or 3 times – I tried to strangle myself because I did not want to live. During my first marriage it was the same things – severe, severe depression.*

TH: *Are you saying that – obviously, you have a history going all the way back to 5, but then it re-surged again after the marriage – was a response to it?*

PT: *It got triggered again.*

TH: *So do you think these things are related – depression, suicidal thoughts, and impotence?*

PT: *I think they are separate issues and the reason is because I have been reading – your book and other stuff. I am a half-baked Psychologist. OK, so during those years of depression I had severe migraines 4–5 times a week.*

The patient reported that a physician friend had recommended Dr. Sarno's (1991, 1999) books a number of years prior to our meeting. As a result of reading these books on the mind-body connection, his migraines had disappeared. He understood that his headaches were triggered by anger at his PhD advisor, who was perceived as pushing his own ambition and agenda on him. He added that this was just like his father, who pushed him to come to the US so that he would look good and could brag to his friends. I decided to use this as an opportunity to test out his capacity to experience the rage directly toward these men.

PT: *My advisor was always pushing his agenda on me – just like my father did.*

TH: *And so your advisor was a stand in for him? You also say you realize you are angry with both of them.*
PT: *Yes.*
TH: *Should we start with your advisor or your father?*
PT: *What do you think?*

Rather than answer the question or simply lob it back at him, highlighting his tendency to behave in a passive, compliant, people-pleasing manner with the therapist was the priority. Again, character defenses must be addressed before specific defenses against specific feelings.

TH: *This is interesting. Is there a tendency for you to be passive and compliant? Because you say, "I didn't want to go to the US. My father wanted it", but I notice you are in the US. He didn't have a gun to your head, so you complied.*
PT: *Right.*
TH: *Here I ask, "where should we start?" and you ask me.*
PT: *GOT IT! Right. I will start with my father. I was always furious with him. Right now I'm furious with him!*
TH: *Something recent?*
PT: *The way he treats my mother. He still abuses my mother now.*
TH: *Physically?*
PT: *Physically, as well as verbally.*
TH: *What's an example of this?*
PT: *An example of physical abuse? I have seen him hitting her when I was a child. I have seen him hitting her now.*
TH: *What's the picture? Where you were and what you actually saw – how he hit her, where he hit her? What exactly happened?*
PT: *There were many times.*

Trying to access feelings in general, without a specific time and incident, rarely goes anywhere. The patient was defending against both his feelings and the specific memories that trigger them. As such, this vagueness needed to be challenged. Initially, the patient used the defense of deference and submissiveness, then resorted to vagueness. Each defense had to be addressed in turn.

TH: *I know, but let's look at a specific example.*
PT: *Well, I will have to think. Well, I do not recollect everything. I just know he's hitting her.*
TH: *Is your mind getting fuzzy? That's something you don't forget. What is happening? Are you getting anxious?*
PT: *No, I am not getting anxious.*

It is important to ascertain whether the apparent collapse of memory is due to overwhelming anxiety or reliance on defenses, as very different interventions would be used in each case. Since he denied anxiety, his defense of forgetting was challenged. His response confirmed that this was an accurate assessment.

TH: *So if you let yourself remember, where would it happen? In the living room or in the kitchen?*
PT: *I see that happen in the kitchen. She's in the corner. He is just going and hitting her.*

In this case, it only took one challenge to his vagueness to produce a specific example. In other cases, defenses can prove more intractable and require significantly more attention.

TH: *Where?*
PT: *On her face. He always hit her on the face.*
TH: *Wow. And you feel angry with him for doing this, yeah?*
PT: *I am angry and scared.*
TH: *But he's not here, so right now?*
PT: *I'm angry.*
TH: *How do you feel it?*
PT: *I have it here* (points to chest).
TH: *What does it feel like in there?*
PT: *I want to hit him.*
TH: *What does it feel like? Do you feel that with heat and power and strength? Is it surging within you?*
PT: *Yes, I feel something here.*

Since this man had a history of acting out feelings as a way to defend against experiencing them, I wanted to make sure he was in touch with the physiological activation of anger before going to the impulse that was being mobilized. While it was understandable that he would have been very frightened by his father's violent behavior as a child in that situation, there is nothing to fear in remembering it as an adult. Fear is a response to a threat to life and limb. In contrast, anxiety is a response to an inner threat. In this case, the threat was facing his own violent and retaliatory impulses.

TH: *How much of the anger that you know you feel toward your father are you feeling right now?*
PT: *I have mixed feelings.*
TH: *Sure, but when you think of him abusing your mother, there's nothing mixed about that is there?*
PT: *No.*

TH: *So how much of the anger you know you have do you let yourself feel?*
PT: *Now I'm not feeling it.*
TH: *So where is it going – because you know you are furious about this.*
PT: *So I am guessing in the body.*
TH: *You guess or you can feel that? We don't want you being a good boy here and going along, saying what you think you are supposed to say.*
PT: *I'm feeling it here in my hands and my arms* (makes fists).
TH: *So if this rage and fury came out of you onto him, to stop him, what do those hands want to do?*
PT: *Just hit him in the face.*
TH: *Hit him how?*
PT: *With my knuckles. Yeah. I'm feeling it in my hands and arms.*
TH: *If all that fury was released through your hand and fists onto him, what do you see happening in your imagination?*
PT: *I just see hitting him* (motions to punch his own face).
TH: *But not you. Do you see that?*
PT: *Right.*
TH: *This is very important. You are the one who gets the headaches, but it's him you want to hit.*
PT: *Yes.*

This patient demonstrated an entrenched pattern of turning angry impulses back on himself, resulting in headaches, hitting himself, and threatening to kill himself. It was essential to spot the process of instant repression as it happened (as when he motioned to punch himself) in order to block it and link this displacement to his symptoms.

TH: *So we want to make sure we face it where it belongs so it doesn't get re-directed. If that were to come out on him, pounding on his head.*
PT: *Yes, I'm just thinking what would happen if I hit him. I would just punch him and punch him – punch his face, punch his temples.*
TH: *And what else, if it all came out and you were going to stop him from beating and abusing your mother?*
PT: *I'm feeling sad as well, and guilty for hitting him. I feel I should not hit him even though what he's doing is wrong.*
TH: *Number one, are you hitting your father?*
PT: *No.*
TH: *So this is where we can see, even to think about it, even to admit there's a part of you that would want to beat the hell out of him – maybe even stop this once and for all.*
PT: *I don't want to go to that extent.*
TH: *But we know you wanted to kill yourself and we can see … so that's for what?*
PT: *Yes, maybe I thought of killing him a couple of times.*

While this patient employed a full roster of formal and tactical defenses, they were not tightly bound. In most cases, one or two rounds of calling the passivity, vagueness, forgetting or denial into question, and these defensive efforts collapsed. Further, new material was revealed, resulting in an increase in the alliance as the resistance fell away.

PT: *Yes, I always wanted him to die.*

TH: *Die how?*

PT: *I just wanted him to die. Yes, and I want him to be dead now.*

TH: *Absolutely. And when you admit this, because he's such a threat to your mother and pain in your neck, that you would want rid of him.*

PT: *Yes.*

TH: *But to really face the part of you that could beat him to death, then other feelings come. Sad feelings and guilty feelings. So, how have you punished yourself for having these feelings and wishes?*

PT: *I just internalize those.*

TH: *Including a death sentence.*

PT: *Right. Yes.*

TH: *As if you had actually committed the crime.*

PT: *Yes.*

TH: *And you're saying, all the back from childhood you wanted rid of this guy but you were the one that would kill yourself. So that is punishment for what crime? For wanting him dead.*

PT: *Right, I wanted him dead.*

TH: *And at the same time there are mixed feelings, sad feelings, and guilty feelings as if there is also some caring for him.*

PT: *I do care for him. I hate him for not being a good husband but as a father he gave me everything, like education. He saved money for my education.*

At this early juncture (this was the first hour of the trial therapy), the therapeutic objective included activating the patient's complex mixed feelings toward others, and then driving home the insight into the pattern of internalization and self-punishment which had been responsible for his suffering. In particular, priority was given to making direct and specific link between his suppressed sadistic impulses and his symptoms. This intervention was designed to turn the ego on the defenses and bolster the alliance.

So far, we had identified two central factors contributing to his symptoms of depression and impotence: (1) internalization of rage toward his father and (2) punishment for guilt over this rage.

Hour 2 – The Plot Thickens

TH: *It sounds like you are saying you are closer to your mother than your father?*

PT: *Oh yes, absolutely. I am much closer to my mother.*

TH: *Are you the oldest?*

PT: *Yes – one younger brother. My brother would stand up against my father always, in the past and in the future. I felt I was a coward. I felt I did not protect my mother, because I was scared of him. I wanted to be a good son.*

TH: *So you really felt torn between them – wanting your father's approval and wanting to protect your mother but watching her get beaten, which is a big load of guilt on you, that you didn't.*

PT: *Yes, that's the guilt I have. I'm here [in the US] because I don't want to be in that house. The culture is different in India. I would have to stay in my parent's house.*

TH: *You didn't want to bring a woman into a house with your father. No way.*

PT: *That's right. Absolutely right. Yes. I did not want that.*

TH: *So then we have to wonder, since you have such heavy guilt that you didn't protect your mother who, let's face it, was your first love, right?*

PT: *My mother is my first love? Of course, yes, yes.*

TH: *And you failed her in your mind and have lots of guilt about that.*

PT: *Yes.*

TH: *So how can you let yourself have a happy marriage and great sex then?*

PT: *Yes. Right.*

TH: *So if you need to punish yourself, in a sense,*

PT: *Yes. So when I fight with my wife now – I don't abuse her physically– but I throw things. I break things.*

TH: *So for sure you are punishing yourself for this anger – either internalizing it with all kinds of symptoms – or acting it out and feeling terrible.*

PT: *Yes. I feel terrible.*

In this vignette, we were examining the conscious guilt he suffered, both because he did not protect his mother and because he had been exposing his wife to traumatic experiences. This was directly connected to his dismal sex life. How could he allow himself to enjoy his wife and have a wonderful sexual life when he had utterly failed to protect his first love? As this was confronted, he looped back to rage at his father and wishing him dead.

PT: *I only think of his death. That's the only way out of this.*

TH: *How do you kill him? How would you triumph, and he goes down?*

PT: *I always think of punching him in the face until he's down. Maybe I thought of choking him.*

TH: *Can you feel that in your hands, the power and strength, because you are practically white knuckled there?*

PT: *Yeah. Grabbing his neck and just strangling him. Maybe that's why I used to strangle myself.*

In this second round of rage toward his father, the patient faced the impulse to punch and choke him to death. This was followed by a spontaneous link between this previously unconscious wish and his suicidal actions as a child, in which he tried to strangle himself. Both the ability to face his own murderous rage and to link this to his previous suicide attempts spoke to his increased capacity, as well as the strength of the unconscious therapeutic alliance (UTA). The fact that ego adaptive capacity can increase dramatically in such a short time (we are still in the first two-hour session) is something many fail to believe is possible. This has more to do with a lack of training in these highly effective techniques than with the reality that deep and lasting change must take a long time to achieve.

Day 2 – Feelings toward His Mother

The patient arrived for the second two-hour session the following day, smiling and looking relaxed.

TH: *Your own thoughts, feelings, and reactions to yesterday?*
PT: *I felt – I felt relaxed. After the session, at the hotel, I was relaxed. It was a good feeling – something light.*
TH: *Yes because you've been living with such a heavy burden.*
PT: *Yes, I was light. I did not think about my father. I was tired. We slept for 2 hours and then went for dinner. I felt light.*
TH: *So you felt lighter and were able to enjoy the time with your wife?*
PT: *Yeah, I did. It was different. It was like meeting her for the first time, maybe*
TH: *Without all these other people in between.*
PT: *It was different.*

Response to intervention is the ultimate assessment tool in our arsenal. While we might assume that a patient with a history of suicidal depression from the age of five would take years to treat, in this case, the patient proved highly motivated and responsive, demonstrating considerable capacity to bear very strong and conflictual feelings. Along with a drastic reduction in his symptoms after the first session, he reported a completely new experience with his wife. Instead of projecting and displacing rage from his father onto her, he was able to see her more clearly, as if for the first time. Furthermore, they enjoyed one another's company and even had a positive sexual encounter. So, even though his sexual life was not a specific or direct focus in our first session, there was significant change in that target symptom. We needed to understand how and why that had taken place. Insight into both the development and relief of symptoms is required for lasting change.

TH: *Your presenting complaint was impotence with your second wife. We didn't talk about it directly, and yet what came up was rage toward your father and feeling trapped in the marriage as you did as a child. What else? Do you see any way in which what we did yesterday is somehow related to sexual difficulties?*

PT: *Do I see they are related? I thought about it but couldn't find any relation. With my ex-wife, most likely it was an excuse that I was depressed all the time, which is partially true but mainly I wasn't interested in her.* (He had married his first wife out of guilt, as he had had sex with her before marriage – something prohibited in his family and by his religious beliefs.)

TH: *You had trapped yourself again, by forcing yourself to do something you didn't want to do out of guilt.*

PT: *Right. More with this wife, I did not get a chance to get to know her. In my perception, it was forced on me, but again, as you mentioned, it was submission, and I didn't stand up for myself. So I should blame myself for that. I cannot connect my rage toward my father, at least not to my ex-wife because it was in my hands, but yeah, with my present wife.*

TH: *And, interestingly, with your first wife, you were able to get erections and penetrate her. You didn't have a lot of desire, but you were able to function, whereas it is different now. Now you can't even do that. We saw how, in the face of your own massive rage toward your father, it is terrifying, and you take a collapsed, impotent position with him.*

PT: *Um hum, um hum, um hum.*

TH: *So this whole thing – you submitting to his choice is also because you are so afraid of your own anger and can't "stand up". Again, what does a penis have to do? Stand up and be erect and strong and so on.*

PT: *Now that I think about it. Because she was chosen by him, that's a way of protesting maybe.*

TH: *That too, but who ends up suffering?*

PT: *Me mainly, and my wife, of course.*

TH: *All this displacement in which he gets off Scott free and all your rage toward him gets turned back on you or displaced onto your wife.*

PT: *True!*

TH: *You've freed yourself from much suffering, like migraines, but it shows up now primarily with women in this triangular situation with your mother and father. You love your mother and want to protect her. To do that you would literally have to kill your father. There is so much sorrow and guilt that you have been nearly paralyzed. Here you are again in another triangle with you, your father, and your wife.*

This material suggested that, in addition to a conflict regarding intense mixed feelings toward his father, a triangular conflict between he, his father, and both his mother and wife emerged as a significant factor involved in his difficulties. The hypothesis that strong mixed feelings toward his mother were also involved had to be tested out.

TH: *And the fact that your mother would come to you and tell you* [what your father was doing] *and that stirs up a lot of feelings too – being put in that impossible position.*

PT: *Yeah, but I still don't get that kind of feeling for my mother.*

TH: *It's much harder to face that you have mixed feelings toward her.*

PT: *Though I will say I wanted her to be dead always.*

Frankly, I was shocked when the patient so readily admitted death wishes toward his mother. This was yet more evidence of the power of the unconscious alliance and its effect of overcoming resistance.

TH: *You did?*

PT: *Yes. Because I saw that was the only way of ending her suffering. Yes, I wish she would be dead so she would be …*

TH: *When do you remember having that wish?*

PT: *That was when I was in India – when, yes, when I was in the USA, I didn't see her suffering. That's the reason I'm in the USA because I cannot see her suffer, but I wanted her to be dead during my teenage years.*

TH: *A huh. So, what's a situation when you remember having those thoughts?*

PT: *Because I saw my father was harassing her and doubting her character. She was a working woman.*

TH: *Where did she work?*

PT: *She had a clerical job so she was doing good, but I could see her suffer emotionally. My father was hitting her, and she had so many health issues because of that. I wished her dead because I had no solution.*

TH: *Because you couldn't bear to witness this and yourself be in such a powerless position.*

PT: *Right.*

TH: *Yesterday you said the only solution would be for your father to die or to kill him to free your mother, but now you are also aware that at times you wished your mother dead – that would be the other way to end this. So how would she die in your fantasy?*

PT: *She would just die. I don't know.*

TH: *Put her out of her misery? How?*

PT: *Because she was so sick. I was like – you know, maybe, OK, she used to travel, and I thought maybe she would have an accident on the train. We have trains and I thought maybe she would die in an accident. I used to be worried and go to the train station to pick her up.*

TH: *Very mixed feelings – wanting to protect your mother and also wanting to be rid of her. So how do you imagine her dying in a train wreck? It's a very painful wish – half of you wanting it, half of you fearing it as you're waiting for her.*

PT: *I don't remember if I wanted her to commit suicide or not. I don't remember that.*

TH: *But it comes to your mind now.*
PT: *Yeah. Yes, because I was always planning suicide!*

Another factor contributing to the patient's symptoms emerged an identification with his suffering mother, in which he was doing to himself what he had wished for her. This was a way to simultaneously spare her and punish himself.

TH: *We can see part of you wishing your mother would kill herself and that would confront or expose your father, that it was clearly his fault, as it was intolerable to live with him.*
PT: *Right.*
TH: *How do you imagine she would kill herself?*
PT: *Just jumping in front of the train.*
TH: *She would be run over by the train?*
PT: *Yes.*
TH: *So how do you see that? The body of your mother on the train tracks?*
PT: *Yeah. I don't know. It was a horrible death (crying). But I wanted her to die.*
TH: *How do you see her body?*
PT: *It's cut (crying). She, she, she did not have a happy life.*
TH: *But then to face that was so intolerable for you – to be exposed to this endless suffering – that you would almost want to push her yourself to get rid of her and this situation. What's this feeling coming up now when you imagine her dead in this horrible way – run over by a train and cut into pieces? How do you see her face?*
PT: *The face of a suffering human being.*
TH: *What's the feeling inside you?*
PT: *I couldn't do anything for her, and I still can't.*
TH: *Part of you wanted to put her out of her misery, and the only way you could see to do that was through death. And to face the part of you that would want to kill the mother who you love. What's the feeling inside of you when you face that? Is it just sorrow and pain or also a guilty feeling?*
PT: *It's sadness, not guilt. Maybe a little happiness that she is dead. It's over. Maybe she'll have a better life next time.*
TH: *What is your belief about that? She'd be in a peaceful place?*
PT: *I think so. Yes, she is a good person. She has never hurt anyone – she has only suffered. I wanted her dead. I couldn't change my father. I still can't change him at 73 years old. I see her now and she's so tired – looks so old.*
TH: *How has this been for you to live with basically death wishes against both of your parents?*
PT: *There was a difference between those two deaths.*
TH: *OK. Tell me. You mean one is a mercy killing in a sense?*
PT: *And one is a murder. Of course, I am not killing her. I am killing him.*

TH: *But it's still your wish.*
PT: *It is my wish. It was my wish. It is my wish.*
TH: *So that feels different to you. But I would imagine that would be a terrible conflict to want to kill the mother you love.*
PT: *Yes but that love is useless if I can't do anything about it. In that sense, maybe my brother loved her more because he stood up, which I don't do.*

Now another triangular conflict between his brother, mother, and himself was revealed.

TH: *Yes. I was thinking about that too – why would you attack your brother for standing up for you? Sounds like you had very mixed feelings about this younger brother showing you up. He took a stand when you didn't, for your mother and against your father.*
PT: *Maybe I was jealous of him. I don't think I'm jealous of him but in my subconscious mind I might be.*

Additional factors contributing to his symptoms continued to be revealed. Massive grief about not being able to protect his mother was accompanied by a wish that she would kill herself – something he had tried to do to himself several times as a child. While I imagined such a wish would evoke guilt, he denied this, stating it was a feeling of intense grief and an anguished sense of helplessness, along with desperate desire to spare her this interminable suffering, that propelled his own suffering. While acknowledging a murderous wish toward his father, which generated guilt, he described his death wish toward his mother as an act of love and mercy. He was of the Hindu faith and believed in the phenomenon of reincarnation. In his mind, death was an avenue to freedom and an act of mercy.

At the end of this session, he reintroduced his brother as another important figure to consider. It is incumbent upon the therapist to be sensitive to cultural and religious differences between patients. It is never our place to question religious beliefs but to understand how they may help or hinder the patient's progress. In this case, he was clear that the death of his mother would be an act of mercy. Clearly, no guilt would be attached to such a wish.

Day 3

PT: *I've been thinking about my brother since our session yesterday, and how I shaped his life. That is killing me. I shaped his childhood by displacing my anger – by hitting him, a person who is loving me and defending me and would take a bullet for me – I abused him, I hit him.*

The UTA was very strong at this point and introduced yet another factor involved in his suffering – guilt about a jealous rage toward his brother was another factor driving his need to kill himself.

PT: *I used to hit him – we used to fight, but the one which bothers me is when he'd come to protect me, then I used to hit him (motioning with his arm).*
TH: *Hit him? Hit him where?*
PT: *On his back. On his back (gasp and sob). It was very painful. I know it was painful for him because I was hitting him with all the force in my body and why was I hitting him?*
TH: *Yes. Exactly.*

The patient went on to detail the ways in which he would provoke children on the school yard to attack him. During such encounters, his brother would often come to his aid. He would then turn on his brother, hitting him and chasing him off, a reaction he found both troubling and completely baffling. Furthermore, he acknowledged that this animosity toward his brother continued into adulthood. For example, his brother asked him for help in relocating to the States. He did not want him to come, and refused to help, with one flimsy excuse after the other.

TH: *So, if you're really honest with yourself, you had very mixed feelings about having him come.*
PT: *I didn't want him to come.*
TH: *And invade your territory.*
PT: *No, I didn't feel that way. No, no, no, I never felt jealous of him for anything.* (Of course, he had admitted being jealous in the session yesterday, so this is simple negation.)
TH: *Even for being born and taking your mother away?*
PT: *Oh, yeah. I don't remember this, but my mother tells me that when he was born and she was in the hospital, I was angry. I was standing at the door, and I was angry so, yes, it's possible, in my subconscious mind, that I was always angry with him.*
TH: *For even existing and taking your mother's attention. You were her first and you had a very special relationship and here comes this competitor. What did she tell you about how you expressed this anger?*
PT: *I was glaring at her and wouldn't go to her for a long time.*
TH: *You were mad at her too. You had her exclusively and then he butts in, so even when he butts in to help, a part of you is so angry that he's interfering, and you want him out.*
PT: *I want him out. I wanted him out. It was like, "This is my fight. Let me fight it."*
TH: *Right.*

PT: *I didn't used to like it. Where I come from, parents and children don't sleep separately. I didn't used to like that he would sleep with my mother. I didn't used to like that much. Yeah. I don't know if that has to do with beating him up.*

TH: *Well, it seems like that came pretty spontaneously. You said, "let me fight my own fight" and realizing that, right from the start, from his birth, you didn't want him around.*

PT: *Jealous. I think, yes, I'm jealous sometimes. I am! And, yes, now thinking back, when he planned to come to the States, maybe I felt threatened. I still do things like tell him that my mother won't make a special meal for him, like she does for me. I do things like that, even now. I was jealous of him – that my father loved him more than me.*

TH: *Angry that he got the love your father withheld from you.*

PT: *He used to tell him he loved him, which he never told me. He said, "You are my life. I can't live without you." He didn't want him to go to the States.*

TH: *So there was a lot of anger and you acted on that jealous and fury by attacking him.*

PT: *Yes, it is, unfortunately, yes. It's hard to acknowledge. But, now I realize I am not responsible for my mother's misery, for what my brother chooses for his life. He has his own free will.*

TH: *You are only responsible for you and how you deal with your feelings and treat others.*

The patient went on to make links between his brother and his wife, seeing that he has competed with her and put her down (calling her stupid, for example), just as he had with his brother. Not only was he jealous of his brother's close relationship to their mother, but with their father as well. As he faced his jealous rage, and his guilt about this rage, he could see how he had tortured himself with an excessive sense of responsibility. The heavy burden of guilt was being lifted. His view of himself and others was being revised accordingly.

PT: *When I see my father's – my dead father's face – I have that, OK, I see a poor man begging for his life. The face I can't explain. He's very poor – like it's not his fault. He has suffered himself as well. That's the face of the suffering man, but then I have this guilt that, whatever good life I have, I am killing this man who helped me.*

TH: *The fact is there are mixed feelings. Even though you are so angry and can hate him at times, you still …*

PT: *I am still happy that he's alive because if he wouldn't be, then I wouldn't have gone past 12th grade.*

TH: *If he had died …*

PT: *I wouldn't have been professionally successful. He was not a good husband or human being, but he made sure that he provided. It's just such mixed feelings and, because of that, I don't want to kill him. But the guilt is that I killed him in my fantasy many times.*

TH: *Have you suffered enough?*

PT: *Yes, I have suffered for my guilt. I am ready to free myself. I'm ready. I'm strong. I'm free.*

In this case, many factors were involved in the creation and maintenance of the patient's symptoms and suffering. He had habitually internalized rage at his father, doing to himself what he had wanted to do to him. This served both a protective function and a punitive one. Much as he hated his father, he also loved him and courted his favor. There was terrific pain and grief over the fact that his father never expressed his love for him. In contrast, his father openly expressed love for his brother, triggering jealousy and rage toward him. He tended to act out this anger at his brother, hitting him in childhood and refusing to help him as an adult. Doing so only increased his sense of guilt.

Finally, he harbored death wishes toward his beloved mother and felt a heavy load of guilt for failing to protect her. With such a heavy burden of guilt upon him, the need to punish himself with symptoms and deprive himself of happiness with his wife could be understood.

The fact that his wife had been chosen by his father was another factor involved in his displaced anger toward her. He tended to be quite stubborn and refused to enjoy the wife his father had chosen for him. Once he faced his rage and guilt about that rage, he was able to meet his wife, "as if for the first time" and to initiate a positive sexual relationship with her. Activating and working through the mixed feelings toward his brother, rather than enacting them with his wife, was another factor involved in resolving these conflicts.

Summary

In this chapter, we have reviewed the concept of multiple causation and detailed cases in which many factors were found to be responsible for the patient's symptoms and suffering. In addition, multiple therapeutic interventions were often required to help patients work through and resolve their difficulties. That said, doing so does not necessarily take months and years. In the case of "The Immigrant," a major resolution was achieved in only six hours of therapy.

Chapter 4

The Repetition Compulsion

Why would a bright and attractive young woman repeatedly rebuff suitable mates and compulsively pursue unavailable and abusive men instead? Why would a talented and educated man interact with superiors in such a way that prompts repeated dismissal from his post? These destructive and repetitive patterns of behavior have confused and vexed therapists since the days of Freud.

In his 1914 paper, "Remembering, Repeating, and Working Through," Freud grappled with these questions in some depth. He suggested several factors contributing to this phenomenon. He discovered that patients tended to repeat what they could not remember, enacting the difficulties they could not report (as they are frequently buried within the unconscious). In other words, patients repeat with the therapist (as well as spouses, bosses, etc.), in the here and now, their unresolved conflicts from the past. While acting out conflicts is understood as a defensive phenomenon, such behavior contains vital expressive elements as well. Freud came to believe that the compulsion to repeat was ultimately an expression of hope and an attempt at mastering, in the present, what was passively experienced in the past. However, without therapeutic intervention, such mastery rarely occurs. Instead, misery is perpetuated. It is up to the therapist to detect these repetitions and help the patient rework rather than repeat them, so that "what went wrong can go right," as Malan put it (personal communication).

As Stark (1994) pointed out, transference phenomena serve both salubrious and destructive purposes.

> That the patient compulsively repeats his past in the present is double-edged. On the one hand, the compulsive repetitions fuel the resistance, fuel the transference. On the other hand, they are the forces that make possible belated master of the early-on environmental failures, mastery achieved by way of working through the resistance, working through the transference.
>
> (p. 10)

DOI: 10.4324/9781003197669-4

In "Mourning and Melancholia," Freud (1917) proposed another factor involved in the repetition compulsion. In addition to an attempt at mastering traumatic experiences, the defense of identification is often involved in this phenomenon. Rather than tolerate all the intense mixed feelings evoked by the loss of loved ones, some patients identify with the lost object and treat themselves the way they were treated. In so doing, the patient staves off grief by continuing the relationship with the lost figure. Unconscious anger toward the lost loved one is frequently involved in such cases. Freud found that patients often identify with the hostile and punitive aspect of the other, as a means of exacting revenge on the part of the self that has come to represent the lost figure.

Freud suggested other, seemingly opposing factors, responsible for the repetition of negative and harmful patterns of behavior, including the death instinct (an innate tendency for all living creatures to return to their original, inorganic state). While the notion of a death instinct did not catch on, the idea that we repeat traumatic interactions in an attempt to master them certainly has. Weiss and his colleagues (1993) have been enthusiastic supporters of this notion – proposing that our patients are highly motivated, albeit unconsciously, to repeat old destructive patterns in the transference in order to have them ameliorated. The therapist's task is to understand and identify a corrective response to the patient's "test," lest he unwittingly confirm and repeat harmful interactions with the patient that only serve to reinforce destructive and limiting beliefs.

Repeating instead of remembering creates resistance. Freud came to realize that bringing all the patient's resistances out into the open – often in the transference – was necessary for their destruction. He wrote, "One cannot defeat an enemy who is absent or not within range" (1914, S.E., XII: 151). But unlike Freud, who increasingly came to rely on a passive approach to such resistance in the therapeutic relationship, Habib Davanloo (1978, 1980, 1990, 2000) advocated a swift and direct approach to resistances in the transference as soon as they become manifest. He was particularly interested in elucidating both formal defenses and those he termed "tactical" (used interpersonally to prevent closeness with the therapist), in order to challenge them and, in so doing, mobilize the patient's previously repressed feelings. In that sense, he considered resistance a "good thing," as it alerts the therapist to the fact that painful and anxiety-provoking feelings are close to the surface. Rather than back off in response to resistance, Davanloo (1990) encouraged therapists to forge ahead and confront resistance head on, knowing that intense and conflictual feelings lay just beneath the surface of the resistance. Completing this process as soon as possible, often in the first encounter with the patient, was found to accelerate and condense the therapeutic process.

Freud believed that only through a full-blown transference neurosis, in which the patient repeats and re-enacts their relationship with an early caretaker in an organized, intense, and consistent fashion with the person of the therapist, could his neurosis be healed. Unfortunately, such transference neuroses often proved difficult to disentangle and resolve. All too often, the analysis became interminable (Freud, 1937). To avoid such difficulties, and streamline the therapeutic process, others (Alexander & French, 1946; Davanloo, 1990) have argued for the avoidance of a wholesale transference neurosis, by bringing feelings toward the therapist into awareness as soon as they were detected. This strategy has proved effective in creating a rapid opening into the unconscious, allowing the therapy to be accelerated, while avoiding the dangers of a transference neurosis (Abbass, Joffres & Ogrodniczuk, 2008, 2009; Davanloo, 1990).

Whereas Freud recommended a stance of "analytic neutrality" in order to allow for a transference neurosis to develop unimpeded, others (Alexander & French, 1946; Davanloo, 1990) have encouraged therapists to abandon therapeutic neutrality. For example, Davanloo emphasized importance of taking a stand *for* openness, honesty, and the courage to face what has been avoided and *against* the resistance that blocks therapeutic action and fuels repeating cycles of suffering. Since resistance will ultimately lead to the defeat of treatment efforts, confronting it head on as soon as it "crystalizes in the transference," fortifies the alliance and speeds the process of healing (Davanloo, 2000). In this way, we are more likely to facilitate a new and corrective experience from the outset of treatment, rather than repeating an old, dysfunctional one (Alexander & French, 1946).

This is often easier said than done, as the patient's pattern of interaction pulls for dysfunctional reactions from others, including the therapist. Fairbairn (1952) and the other object relation theorists (Clark & Scharff, 2014) were among the first to conceive of this "compulsion to repeat" as a result of internalized early relationships. Mitchell and Black (1996) summarized the pattern:

> Each of us shapes his relationships according to the patterns internalized from his earliest significant relationships. The modes of connection with early objects become the preferred modes of connection with new objects … New love objects are chosen for their similarity to bad (unsatisfying) objects in the past; new partners are interacted with in a way that provokes old, expected behaviors; new experiences are interpreted as if they fulfilled old expectations.
>
> (pp. 121–22)

In his theory of cyclical psychodynamics, Wachtel (1977) expanded upon this view by including a more interpersonal perspective: people elicit specific behavior from their intimates – even behaviors uncharacteristic of those people – that allow for their own repetitions to be re-enacted on a continual basis. Thus, the repetition compulsion has both intrapsychic and interpersonal components, and the pull for the therapist to be drawn into them is strong.

Finally, the patient's need to suffer due to unconscious guilt is an additional factor that must be considered in the development and perpetuation of the repetition compulsion. If the patient is driven to suffer by unconscious forces, therapy will be no exception. In fact, the need to suffer and remain ill will completely derail treatment efforts if not detected and confronted as soon as it becomes apparent.

Many of our patients have managed to defeat countless therapists. It is an error to assume that all these therapists were incompetent and that you can be successful without the patient's active participation. Reigning in our own omnipotent fantasies is required. Instead, a procedure labeled "the head on collision" (Davanloo, 1999), in which the patient is confronted with the ways in which his defenses and resistances have, and will continue to, undermine treatment if not abandoned, is often necessary in such intransigent cases. In addition to confronting such destructiveness, an appeal must be made to the healthy part of the patient, longing to connect with the therapist in a constructive manner in order to free himself of the need from suffering. While demonstrating the greatest sympathy and respect for the patient's "true self," we must call his resistances into serious question. Focusing on the conflict between the healthy part of the patient seeking freedom and the part of him clinging to defenses that fortify resistance is required in order to create an intrapsychic crisis and precipitate an opening of the unconscious, where healing can take place.

It is the eventual exhaustion of all the defenses, leading the patient to experience her underlying feelings, that leads to the "unlocking of the unconscious" and the end of the repetition compulsion. Davanloo (1990) wrote:

> Where a therapist has achieved a major breakthrough with a resistant patient, this has almost invariably followed a passage in which the patient has been confronted with his feelings in the transference and has been able to experience and acknowledge them ... the patient becomes angry within an atmosphere in which he senses, both consciously and unconsciously, that the therapist is directing him towards his most painful buried feelings out of a genuine and compassionate concern, a determination not to spare him pain but to make him face it, with the sole purpose of freeing him from the self-defeating patterns that have spoiled his life for so many years. The patient's unconscious will respond by revealing in depth some of the feelings, situations, and events that have led to his neurosis.
>
> (pp. 7–8)

Davanloo stressed the importance of "the systematic analysis of the transference," a process of repeatedly connecting feelings, anxiety, and defenses (the triangle of conflict) in the transference to previously unconscious feelings, memories, anxiety, and defenses from the patient's past and current life (triangle of person). Helping the patient see his role in perpetuating his suffering by repeating dysfunctional patterns of relating is the first step in altering these destructive patterns.

Once the patient discovers the link between the unresolved past and his current feelings toward and perception of the therapist, distinctions are made. The patient is urged to do something different in the here and now. Feeling and reflecting are not enough to create lasting change. Insight must be accompanied by new and constructive action.

It bears repeating that this work, done from the moment these patterns are in evidence in the transference, is key to avoiding a full-blown transference neurosis which can be difficult, if not impossible, to resolve.

The Woman Who Couldn't Love Her Daughter

This 40-year-old married mother of three came for help, having experienced a panic attack and ensuing anxiety over the previous six months. She had recently been recruited to join a prestigious law firm and was invited to a special partner's dinner, where spouses were expected to attend. For reasons she couldn't understand, she had a strong inclination to leave her husband at home. She overrode this impulse and had him join her, but at dinner was seized with intense anxiety and fled to the bathroom, where she cried uncontrollably for some time. She was baffled by her own reaction and decided to pursue treatment in order to get to the bottom of this.

When asked what she made of the incident, she said, "I wasn't proud of him," mentioning, in contrast, how proud she was of an ex-boyfriend. It turns out that her husband had a pattern of ignoring her and refusing to talk when he was upset about something. As it happened, he hadn't been speaking to her for several days prior to the partner's dinner.

As we began to explore feelings toward her husband, she became anxious and disconnected, relying on the defenses of intellectualization and rumination. This lent further support for the notion that an intensification of such feelings was the trigger to her symptoms. In addition, she mentioned feeling as if she was "outside of her body," suggesting a kind of depersonalization when extremely anxious. Such a reaction indicated that anxiety was over the optimal threshold and needed to be downregulated before therapy could proceed apace. Focusing on the actual experience of anxiety in the body proved very useful in lowering high levels of anxiety. Once anxiety returned to an optimal level, a cognitive review of the process was necessary for working through to take place.

As we examined the patient's tendency to focus on positive feelings, to the exclusion of pain and rage, she reported that her husband is kind and funny but has a temper. He lashes out verbally and even shouts "Shut up!" to the kids, which she "doesn't like." When pressed to experience her feelings toward him in this regard she said, "I want to shout back," jumping right over her feelings to the impulse.

In contrast to the shouting going on in her own home, she revealed that her parents rarely spoke, and considered any expression of strong feeling embarrassing, and something to be avoided at all cost. Quite spontaneously, she noticed that she had been refusing to speak to her father, much as her husband refused to speak to her. Avoidance and concealment had become prominent features in her own life. In fact, she had lied to her husband about our session, saying she had a business meeting to attend. She went on to acknowledge the ways in which she had been distancing from her husband, especially in the past six months. "I have a bigger part in this than I saw before," she realized. We could already identify repetitive and destructive patterns in evidence. Rather than deal with her feelings toward her father, she has been identifying with him and repeating his pattern of emotional distancing with both him and her husband.

As these patterns and their consequences were elucidated, she decided to face and experience her true feelings, instead of avoiding them in ways that promoted disconnection from herself and her husband. We returned to the evening of the dinner. She was able to feel an enormous anger welling up within her as she imagined riding with him on the subway. Initially, she felt anxious, tense, and shaky but then experienced her underlying rage, with an impulse to push him out onto the train tracks. Seeing him splayed out on the tracks evoked deep pain and regret, along with loving feelings and a desire for closeness. Her anxiety disappeared (as often happens quite dramatically after the forbidden impulses are experienced directly) and she experienced deep sadness about the distance in relationship to her husband.

Following the breakthrough of mixed feelings toward her husband, a link to her father emerged. About 12 years prior to our meeting, the patient had been living with her father for a short time while renovations to her apartment were taking place. She went out with friends one evening and, having had a bit to drink, decided to stay the night rather than drive home. When she returned the next day, her father greeted her at the door, declaring, "You had better find somewhere else to live." Clearly, he had a habit of dealing with his own feelings of anger and jealousy by distancing. She got in touch with the enormous pain and anger this evoked, but had never been previously experienced.

This first session proved very helpful to the patient. She was able to make sense of her symptoms and understand her own contribution to the distance in both her marriage and in relation to her father.

In the second session, the patient was pensive, having had many memories of growing up in a home where "we were never allowed to be angry." In contrast, she had made a concerted effort to accept and support her children in having all their feelings. Her children were close, in contrast to she and her siblings, who acted out against each other (hitting each other and throwing things, punching holes in the wall) and were often sent to their separate rooms as punishment. Nothing was ever sorted out or resolved. Her parents considered them all "hopeless."

Both parents were busy working, her mother as a medical professional and her father as an engineer. Even when at home, her mother was often involved with paperwork and clearly prioritized career over family. As the patient reported this material, a headache surfaced – indicating a rise of feeling toward her mother that was being internalized.

Session #2

TH: *You end up with a headache, but we have to wonder how you feel toward your mother for being so unavailable. Even when she was home, she was busy with paperwork.*

PT: *I feel sad. I wish she had wanted us.*

TH: *It is sad, but what about the feeling toward her for withholding her love and attention?*

PT: *I didn't want her to come home. She interfered with our happiness. We much preferred being home with my Dad. That reminds me – we were actually happy when they divorced, and she moved out.*

TH: *So, you got your wish – to be rid of your mother and have your father to yourself. How old were you?*

PT: *17 or 18.*

TH: *How did you imagine getting rid of her?*

PT: *I would rather have someone warm and loving. Actually, my father's mother was an important figure in my life. She lived next door and we were welcome any time. That was a place where I felt loved and accepted.*

TH: *You didn't want the mother you had and were happy to be rid of her.*

PT: *She was happy to leave. This is crazy, but I actually went after her. Somehow, I was afraid she would be lonely. Little did I know she actually had another man already. Again, I was in the way, and she didn't want me there with her. I distinctly remember one evening, as I was washing the dishes, I thought, "What is the point?" and left.*

TH: *You tend to go to action without letting yourself feel and accept what is going on within you. Even though you wanted rid of her, you chased after her. You didn't let yourself have what you wanted – to be alone with your Dad – and went to live with her. Then you got fed up and left, but what about your feelings toward her?*

PT: *Now I feel a kind of tightness in my stomach, though my headache is gone!*

TH: *Let's see how you feel toward her rather than filling yourself with anxiety.*
PT: *Yes, I was angry with her.*
TH: *How do you experience that inside?*
PT: *Some tension in my stomach but now I feel a power and strength coming up and into my arms and hands.*
TH: *Your hands are in a fist.*
PT: *Yes, I am really angry and see myself there with her in the kitchen. Actually, I was cleaning up because she had kicked me out of her room, where I went for some affection. I asked if I could lie down next to her, and she said no. I could just punch her – actually I feel like choking her. I just want her out. I would punch her and choke her and jump on her – just choke her until (big sigh).*
TH: *What is coming up? What do you see?*
PT: *I see her dead face. This is strange. I'm not so much sad that she's dead but that I never had her in the first place. I am sick of going to people who aren't available and getting rejected. I suddenly feel this impulse in my leg just to kick her out of the house. I don't even want to touch her. I wish someone else would take care of it.*

The patient was seeing her role in perpetuating the cycle of distance and suffering in her relationships that has previously alluded her. She repeatedly pursued those who were unavailable for an emotional connection – banging her head against the wall, as it were. As she faced these feelings, her headache vanished, and she was able to view her history from a new perspective.

TH: *Who?*
PT: *My father. Yes, he can do it.*
TH: *Interesting.*
PT: *Yes, I am angry he didn't take care of this earlier and that we had to grow up with a mother who was so rejecting. Now I understand why I am so upset with my Dad. I am relieved to be feeling this and understanding it all.*
TH: *Tell me what you understand.*
PT: *I have been really angry with both of them – with my mother for being so cold and distant and with my father for keeping her around all that time. But now I see that I wanted him to get rid of her a long time ago. When she finally left, I was relieved but went to live with her! I turned everything around – wouldn't let myself stay with my Dad but went to take care of her. It's pretty crazy but I can see that I felt guilty about getting my wish and did the exact opposite of what I wanted. Is that what I'm doing with my husband now?*
TH: *We'll explore that next time.*

The patient came into the next session reporting massive relief after the previous session. She reported sitting quietly for quite a while after the meeting, allowing herself to feel the enjoyment of being alive, present, and connected to all her feelings. She went home excited to speak to her husband about what she was discovering, and became very angry when he made it clear he didn't want to hear about it. She caught herself in the old pattern of wanting to withdraw in the face of her anger, but refused to do so this time. She remained present throughout the evening and then he came around, apologizing and asking her to tell him more. Then, a new problem surfaced.

Session #3

PT: *Somehow my two-year-old seemed to notice that I was more present and connected. For some reason I haven't been able to feel very attached to her. I feel terrible about it and don't really understand it, but it's always been that way.*

Up until now, the only problems the patient mentioned were anxiety, panic, and depression, in relation to her husband. As often happens, once the defenses have been relinquished and the unconscious is open, other conflicts and concerns emerge.

TH: *Since her birth or even before? Did you want another child?*

PT: *I absolutely did but – I feel guilty even saying this – my first thought was, "She's not mine." She didn't look like me.*

TH: *Didn't look like you?*

PT: *My other children are fair like me, but she was dark – had dark hair.*

TH: *Dark hair?*

PT: *The whole birth was horrible. The midwife was a robot – she was very strict and demanding and offered no support. She kept saying, "I need you to turn around" –"I need this and that." I was just trying to block her out. "It's not about you!" Oh my, I just realized she had dark, short hair – like my mother!*

By listening to the specifics and reflecting them back to her, the patient made her own link between this dark-haired baby, the midwife, and her mother.

TH: *Now you are starting to see a link between the midwife and your mother – these dark-haired women who are strict and demanding, while devoid of warmth. And the dark-haired baby who reminds you of them.*

PT: *Yes, I was so angry with that horrible midwife. I remember this so strongly – suddenly I had the thought, "I will fall out of the bed, right on the baby." The baby would die. I couldn't figure that out.*

TH: *We see the link between forbidden anger and your tendency to shut down, withdraw and create distance. We also see a link between this buried anger toward the midwife and your mother with your daughter. You have been distanced from her too. Underneath the distancing is anger and a wish to be rid of her that got displaced onto the baby. You wanted to kill her or choke your mother, knock her down and kick her out the door, but thought of throwing yourself on the ground and kill the baby instead.*

PT: *You're right. On top of it, I was angry with my husband at the same time. He was having a hard time at work and prioritized that over our family – just like my mother!*

TH: *And, again, you swallowed that anger and distanced yourself. Where does that anger go? Sometimes it goes back on you with headaches, anxiety, and so on. Here we see it got displaced onto your baby.*

PT: *(crying) It is so clear now.*

TH: *How are you feeling?*

PT: *I am so profoundly relieved to understand all this. It is sad but also a relief. Now I feel really guilty about my poor daughter. I haven't been there for her. I have shut her out as my mother shut me out. This is awful. She is lovely – more quiet and fragile than the other two. She is so clever and was an early talker. I remember a recent time when we were alone together. She took my hand and said, "Mommy, you are my best friend." (Patient weeps.)*

This response to intervention highlights the vital importance of understanding the material that emerged following the experience of previously avoided feelings. Being able to specifically understand the mechanisms responsible for her detachment from her daughter, and the repetition of a pattern of withdrawal in her family of origin, was vital to the healing process. She could see the repetitive pattern and wanted to interrupt it.

Session #4

PT: *The last session was really important. How strange that I never saw it before. As soon as I saw my daughter with the dark hair, I associated her with my mother and rejected her on some level. Then something else came to me after that session – that I had a kindergarten teacher I loved very much. She was blond and warm and kind – nothing like my dark-haired mother. I wanted her to be my mother. It was such a strong wish. I feel it now! I thought I had the wrong mother. I wanted to go home with her, not my mother. Of course, I kept that a secret.*

The patient's unconscious was wide open, and the alliance was promoting deep healing and profound connections between the present and the past.

TH: *Keeping both the wish for a warm, loving mother and the part of you that wanted to be rid of your mother and replace her, secret.*

PT: *I just realized now that wanting another mother and wanting another daughter – or feeling "No, that's not my daughter," and "No, you're not my mother," are connected. This is actually one of my strongest memories, but again, I had to keep it a secret. To be honest, I didn't want another daughter – I already had two. I wanted a son and was disappointed, but felt I had to be grateful – "she's healthy, who cares about gender?" There was no room for my disappointment.*

TH: *All these feelings are understandable and cause no problems, but your anxiety and guilt about these wishes and feelings – keeping it tightly bound and secret – has wreaked havoc.*

PT: *Secrets! You know what? My father only found out that his father wasn't his father when he got sick a few years ago and his mother finally told him. Again, we only talked about feeling grateful for the information and never talked about these other feelings.*

More memories and connections were revealed, allowing the patient to deepen her understanding of herself, and a pattern of emotional distance and secrets keeping that went back generations. These patterns are often repeated from one generation to the next. In this case, the patient was determined to put a stop to it, lest she pass it on to her own children.

TH: *How has all this secrecy affected you?*

PT: *Now I see how unfair this is to my darling daughter. She is so lovely. She doesn't deserve it! Something has really changed with her. I held her a lot and she was so responsive. I feel normal – it's such a relief!*

TH: *Dealing with these feelings and wishes openly and honestly has freed you up to be more real, present, and connected with your daughter.*

PT: *You know – this is really strange – my other two daughters are pretty easy going and independent but this one has always wanted to be close to me. She doesn't want a substitute – but I did!*

TH: *How are you making sense of this?*

PT: *I didn't want my mother to be my mother. I wanted a substitute – my lovely kindergarten teacher. I now understand I felt really guilty about that. Maybe I wouldn't let myself be chosen by my daughter. It's almost as if I wanted her to accept a substitute.*

TH: *As if, out of guilt and a need to suffer, you would have to deprive yourself of that wonderful closeness you always wanted.*

PT: *I feel so much better about it – like it's OK. I feel so much closer to my daughter now, though it's impossible with my mother. About 5 years ago I tried to open up to her to see if we could forge a relationship as adults. She said, "You come along and expect me to fix you."*

TH: *Wow – what kind of feelings does that evoke?*

PT: *It's very painful and infuriating but I can somehow let it be. I have done all I can and it's just not possible. But it is possible for me to have a close relationship with my own children – also with my father and husband.*

Being able to accept the reality of who her mother is and is not, along with her true feelings toward her, was freeing. Not only could she accept that she would not achieve the kind of closeness she wanted with her, but that she could have it with her daughter. Rather than repeating the painful past, he was creating a new future.

Session #5

PT: *This process is amazing. I am so glad I came to see you. I have absolutely fallen in love with my daughter. She runs to me now – "Mommy, Mommy." She is such a gift. I also feel much closer to my husband, having been able to talk to him about wanting a much closer relationship, and how my tendency to distance when angry is affecting us. It's interesting – with both my daughter and husband – when I open up, they do too, and we are closer than ever. Obviously, my husband wasn't talking to me either, but he's really coming around. That said, I am still having issues with my father.*

Wonderful as these changes were to hear, research suggests that a deep understanding of how they have been achieved is essential for sustained change. Given this, I inquired about her understanding of what promoted this level of change.

TH: *What is happening there?*
PT: *I'm not even sure I want to be closer to him. I'm strangely comfortable with the distance. We are very civil and friendly on a superficial level. He is quite involved with my children, but there is an undertone of criticism – the sense that I am always wrong somehow, that he owns the truth, and I am being difficult.*
TH: *Let's see how it's come to that, because initially you were Daddy's girl.*
PT: *But then he asked me to leave.*
TH: *And ever since …*
PT: *Well, even before. I had this wonderful boyfriend, but his father was in jail for some sort of white-collar crime. My father never gave him a chance, but made it clear he didn't like him. He was the love of my life and would do anything for me, but my father undermined the relationship and kept filling me with doubts.*

This new material shed light on the opening statement in the first session, in which the patient said she didn't feel proud of her husband, as she had a previous boyfriend. These memories provided information on what happened in that relationship, and helped us understand why it would be triggered by difficulties in her current marriage.

TH: *It sounds like your father had some feelings about you being in love.*

PT: *It was my first serious relationship. My Dad was still single. Maybe he was jealous. Somehow realizing this is a relief. It's not my problem. Yes, the trouble with my father started then.*

TH: *You have a lot of feelings toward your father for interfering in that relationship.*

PT: *Yes, I feel angry with him but also angry with me for doing what he expected me to do. My body is shaking as I say it.*

TH: *How do you feel this anger at him?*

PT: *It's in my fists again.*

TH: *What do those fists want to do?*

PT: *He was so accepting of me as a child, but not as a young woman. He got angry with me for going out and just showed me the door! I am so angry. He acted poorly but it was as if I was the problem.*

Our time ran out before we were able to fully explore all the feelings toward her father.

Session #6

PT: *I feel such relief since the last session. Now I understand what was happening between me and my father. The tension is gone and so is the guilt. He sees me as difficult, but I don't have to go along with that and agree.*

TH: *Somehow facing your feelings toward your Dad, and understanding his toward you, has shifted something.*

In addition to distinguishing past from present, the patient was increasingly able to distinguish her own sense of self from the opinions (and projections) of others.

PT: *Yes. We had a family gathering over the weekend, and I wondered if I would want more closeness with him, as I have with my husband and daughter, but I didn't. A while back I sent him a letter, but he only acted confused and, again, indicated that I am impossible.*

TH: *What is your feeling toward him? He has been distancing and pushing you away for many years.*

PT: *I'm really annoyed with him. He doesn't listen.*

TH: *How have you been dealing with those feelings?*

Making sure the patient understands own defensive patterns, rather than simply focusing on the experience of feelings, seems essential for deep and lasting change to take place.

PT: *By shutting down and rejecting him. Now I realize it's a big loss and I am angry.*

I am doing to him what he did to me. It's like tit for tat.

TH: *You are acting it out in a way that is destructive, wouldn't you say?*

PT: *Yes. I don't want to be like him.*

TH: *Let's see how you feel that anger inside.*

PT: *I am really boiling. I could punch him right in the face.*

TH: *What else?*

PT: *I push him down and then out to door so hard that he falls on his back. He banged his head looks like a little helpless child.*

TH: *What feeling does that evoke?*

PT: *Satisfaction. I am actually still angry and want to kick him quite a lot.*

TH: *Then what?*

PT: *I want to leave him alone and stranded – just like he did to me.*

TH: *That is what you've done – closed the door on him.*

PT: *Now I feel sad. I really miss him. We were so close. At the same time, I can feel that I wouldn't want him to know how painful this has been for me. That would give him satisfaction.*

TH: *You seem to be engaged in a silent battle of wills and trying to keep the upper hand.*

PT: *That is so childish.*

TH: *What is the price you pay?*

PT: *It's not just with him but I have been doing this same thing with others. When I am hurt and angry – distancing and pretending I don't care, and they can't get to me.*

TH: *It must be lonely.*

PT: *Not so much these days, as I feel really close with my husband and kids, as well as my sisters. The fact is you can't get blood from a stone. My father was close to me when I was a child when he was in charge. He's never been able to have a real relationship with me as an adult. Suddenly I can feel for my mother and what it must have been like for her to bang her head against the wall with him.*

TH: *How is that?*

PT: *My father hated that she was independent – that she worked and had her own car. The same thing happened with me. When I started to have my own life, he got angry. Before that, but after the divorce, he took me on a holiday to Europe. Now it seems kind of creepy to me. We were like an old married couple. I don't want to be his wife!!*

These perceptions of her parents constituted a significant revision from her previous view of them, in which her mother was considered cold-hearted and her father a long-suffering saint. By facing and experiencing her mixed feelings toward them, each became a three-dimensional figure with both laudable and infuriating aspects of their personalities. These revised views of self and other are a hallmark of successful therapies.

TH: *What do you want?*

PT: *I want him to be my father and a grandfather to my children. I can really appreciate him in that role. It's sad I have had to detach so much and this all surprises me a bit. I used to think my Dad was great and my mother was cold as ice, but now I see it differently. He was no angel, and she wasn't all bad.*

TH: *That seems important.*

PT: *Yes. I also wanted to tell you that when I went to pick up my daughter from day care the other day, they said, "It's clear you two are especially close." Everyone can see it and I am so happy about it.*

TH: *You can't go back and re-do your childhood, but you can do it differently now with your own children.*

PT: *Yes indeed.*

Last Session

PT: *I am just amazed at what's happened between me and my daughter. I have found so much love, with her and my husband too. I came here because of that panic attack at the party but got so much more out of this than I ever imagined.*

TH: *That is wonderful.*

PT: *I was thinking about my father yesterday and what happened between us. When he asked me to move out, something broke. Both my parents left me because I was "too difficult," and they gave up. There is deep pain and grief about this. It's almost like I had agreed with them that I was the problem. And it's really not true. I just had one of those 360 evaluations at work and my ratings for interpersonal relating are off the charts. It's not just me, but how I reacted to their criticism and rejection. It really helps to understand that they had problems and limitations too. It's funny but I have no burning need to tell them all this. I know it and feel it's all straightened out within me. I can accept them as they are – and accept me! I really feel happy about that.*

TH: *You are no longer living out their perceptions of you or unconsciously repeating these patterns with your own husband and children.*

PT: *I don't need their approval anymore. At the same time, it is sad that my Dad is so much better with kids than with adults. It was so helpful to feel all the pain and anger that was there. I was just giving him the cold shoulder. It all makes so much sense now. In a funny way, I am even optimistic about my father. If I no longer need him to be something he isn't, I can accept him and feel peaceful about it all. I am actually looking forward to Christmas together. I really appreciate how great he is with my kids.*

TH: *You've done some really hard work here – facing intense mixed feelings that were really scary and guilt inducing – toward your husband, daughter, mother, and father. In so doing, your perspective in it all has been altered in such a way that seems to give you freedom and a sense of peace.*

PT: *If I hadn't come here and done this work, I would still be distant from my husband and subtly rejecting of my daughter. I have made connections I simply never saw before and understand myself, and what happened, so clearly. I can accept it all and don't need to blame anybody.*

This point can't be emphasized strongly enough. All too often therapists collude in the patient's vilification of parents, blaming them for their own difficulties, even into their 60s and 70s! This is not only corrosive to their relationships, but undermines the development of the patient as an autonomous self. In this case, helping the patient accept responsibility for her own feelings, and how they have been handled, enhanced her sense of mastery and competence, while promoting compassion for self and others. Furthermore, it enabled her to interrupt the repetition compulsion and forge a new future in alignment with her own feelings and wishes.

Relationships were no longer an all or nothing proposition (like it or leave it) but nuanced and, inevitably, a mixed bag. She was able to choose what relationships to invest in, like those with her husband and daughter, while pulling back from relationships that offered no mutuality and reciprocity. The need to compulsively pursue the unavailable one had been removed and replaced with something far healthier.

TH: *That's really wonderful.*

PT: *It is. Thank you so much. I am happy but sad at the same time to say goodbye to you. You have really helped me. I felt like such a mess when I first started seeing you.*

TH: *I never experienced you that way. You were incredibly open and responsive – a real pleasure to work with. I feel lucky to have had the chance to get to know you.*

PT: *That really touches me. Now I am crying. It's so moving – to know I can get close and be understood and connect.*

This patient had been repeating a pattern of shutdown and withdrawal that was characteristic of her family of origin. In our very first session, she was able to see how she was repeating that pattern in relationship to her husband and later with her daughter. Once she experienced her own feelings about having been treated in such a dismissive manner, she shifted from avoidance to open expression and connection. As a result, not only did she get relief from her symptoms but healed her relationships as well.

It should be emphasized here that the driving force in the repetition of a generational pattern of emotional distance was attributable to reliance on a number of defenses against anxiety-provoking and guilt-laden feelings promoted and reinforced by her parents. "Trauma" is not passed down from one generation to the next, but habitual patterns of response to the intense emotions triggered by traumatic events often are.

A Woman Abused

A 50-year-old mother of four sought intensive psychotherapy in order to get to the bottom of self-defeating pattern of behavior with men, as well as a long-standing and pervasive tendency to isolate herself and keep an emotional distance from everyone. She had been separated from an abusive husband for four years but was unable to "pull the plug" and get divorced. In so doing, she realized she was remaining tied to him in some way, despite her conscious wish to be done with him. Inquiry revealed that she had suffered significant and repeated physical and psychological abuse at the hands of her father, who was also extremely violent toward her mother and siblings. It was clear to her that she had repeated her mother's pattern in this regard and was highly motivated to put a stop to it once and for all. The only difference between herself and her mother, prior to treatment, was in regard to the protection of children. When her husband started to lash out at them physically, she had him removed from the home and obtained a restraining order. In contrast, her mother actively undermined protective efforts and clung to her abusive husband.

In addition to suffering abuse at the hands of others, the patient reported long-standing depression, accompanied by an ingrained tendency to blame herself for sins of the other. We will begin with the first session, when we focused on an example of abuse at the hands of her husband.

Session #1

PT: *Oh, one of the worst is when I was pregnant with our fourth. He didn't want the child and beat me, kicking me in the stomach.*

TH: *How do you feel toward him?*

PT: *I feel heat and energy rising up – then I feel all tense. When I feel angry, I bang things or slam doors or stomp my feet like a toddler.*

TH: *Trying to get rid of it and protect him – you redirect it, but if that came out at him, in your imagination, if all that rage, energy, and heat come out of you onto him, what would happen?*

PT: *I would punch him.*

TH: *Where?*

PT: *On the chest – banging on him.*

TH: *What else? This is a lifetime of rage, isn't it?*

PT: *I haven't thought about it, though I know it's there.*

TH: *Where does it go then?*

PT: *Back on top of me and my already stressed life (laughs).*

TH: *That isn't funny though.*

Rather than simply press for the experience of rage here, identifying the defenses she has habitually employed against it was an essential prerequisite.

In addition to seeing clearly how she has avoided this rage, feeling the impact of such avoidance is a key element of change. As long as she was laughing off her own abusive and neglectful treatment of herself, therapeutic progress would stall.

PT: *I know.*

TH: *You protect him and turn it back on you with "I am silly. I am stupid." and such. But the rage is toward him. I am not suggesting you do this, but to honestly face what it wants to do to him.*

PT: *I'd kill him.*

TH: *How?*

PT: *(sigh) Every punch I got, given back. The same with my Dad.* (I heard the link but chose not to pursue it until after we were done with her husband.)

TH: *Where do you go for him?*

PT: *Not just his chest but his hair, his face, kick him in the balls. He kicked me when I was pregnant and broke my ribs, but I didn't tell anyone.*

TH: *This is payback – retaliatory rage – give it back to him with punching and kicking. Do you beat him to death?*

PT: *Yes, I am feeling it in my hands. I see him in the kitchen and me doing it.*

TH: *How does he die?*

PT: *(sigh) I haven't seen him die yet. I've hurt him but he's not dead.*

Since the patient had made it clear that her wish was to kill her husband, it was necessary to continue with the fantasy until it reached that end. As these vignettes illustrate, it is inevitable that anxiety and defenses will emerge as previously avoided feelings breakthrough the resistance. Working and re-working the triangle of conflict (Chapter 1, Figure 1.1) is often necessary in order to clarify the relationship between forbidden feelings, the anxiety they generate, and the defenses that have blocked access to the patient's true feelings.

TH: *Could you kill him with kicks and punches or would something else be required?*

PT: *(laugh) I am looking at the frying pan and the knives in the kitchen.*

TH: *Is the laugh from anxiety or is there some sense of satisfaction?*

PT: *It's satisfaction, but there is sadness as well – that this is what he brought me to.*

TH: *How do you kill him and protect yourself and your children?*

PT: *Keep hitting him with the frying pan.*

TH: *Where?*

PT: *In the head.*

TH: *What happens to his head?*

PT: *It bleeds, and it would explode.*

TH: *What's the picture? If you look into his face and eyes.*
PT: *I check that he's breathing. I made eye contact with him twice – looking into his face to see if he was dead, both times he tried to commit suicide.*

This was a very important moment and illustrates the fact that these "fantasies" are always tied in some way to reality. The patient was not making this up, but was remembering wishes and events that had taken place in the past. It turns out that her husband, apparently overcome with guilt about having tried to kill their baby, made a serious suicide attempt after the baby died. The patient was remembering how he looked when she found him, nearly dead after an overdose.

TH: *Clearly that memory right now lets us know that you wanted him dead.*
PT: *Yet I saved him.*
TH: *Exactly – as if you would have been the one who killed him. What did you see?*
PT: *The whites of his eyes – no movement.*
TH: *Is that the same thing you saw when you imagined bashing his head in with the frying pan?*
PT: *Yes. My sister told me I should have waited a few more minutes before going to the house. I should have let him go. Sometimes I feel I should have let him go.*
TH: *How do you feel when you see him dead now?*
PT: *Relieved. He won't be there to torment us anymore because he torments us still with texts begging to come back.*
TH: *There is a restraining order. Why is he contacting you?*
PT: *I can't block him – it's in me.*

There was clearly an unconscious reason she had remained tied to a man she so desperately wanted out of her life. This material suggested that guilt over her murderous rage was at least one factor driving her need to keep him on as a kind of torturer in her life. Exposing the guilt and replacing the need to be punished with compassion and freedom was the immediate therapeutic goal.

TH: *Let's understand this. A big part of you wants him dead and out of your life but you go overboard the other way. Why would you do that? Let's look at how you feel when you see him dead.*
PT: *I feel responsible and also sad and sorry for him.*
TH: *So if you had actually done it, how would you feel?*
PT: *Relief but also guilt. Guilt.*
TH: *How do you punish yourself?*
PT: *By keeping in contact and allowing it.*
TH: *In a weird way you use him to punish you because of this guilt.*

PT: *Right. Right.*

There are many ways in which self-punishment can manifest. Sometimes, the patient directly harms herself with cutting, starvation, and substance abuse, while at other times patients employ other people to use and abuse them. Women in abusive relationships will not be able to sever ties with their abusers until they free themselves from the need to be punished for their retaliatory rage.

TH: *Does the punishment fit the crime?*
PT: *No. I didn't kill him. The punishment doesn't fit the crime.*
TH: *Yet you've been living a life sentence – not freeing yourself.*
PT: *I am still tied to him.*
TH: *Again, you employ him as your prison guard. Is that what you want?*
PT: *No. Not at all.*

Since the patient had experienced mixed feelings toward her husband and could clearly see that she had been punishing herself for murderous wishes, we returned to the link she had made earlier with her father. Getting to the source of the conflicts that were being repeated was necessary to resolve it.

C-P Link

TH: *Earlier you made a link between your husband and your father. When you were in touch with that rage toward Thomas did you get any images of your father?*
PT: *Yes. I'm the only one in the family that keeps in touch with him.*
TH: *So it's the same dynamic of caring for the perpetrator, but if you face your rage toward him, when did you feel that?*
PT: *When he hit my mother. Dad used to hit us with sticks and canes. I see myself with a baseball bat and let him see how it feels to be hit with a stick.*
TH: *Where do you go for him?*
PT: *Body, arms, everywhere he hit us, in the head. I went to school with a black eye.*
TH: *Why wasn't he put in jail?*
PT: *He always got away with it. My Mom's family wanted us to leave and report him, but she begged them not to.*
TH: *You must have feelings toward her too.*
PT: *I am angry with her but it's so hard. I love her too. Everyone loves her. She is so kind.*
TH: *If we stay with your father, what do you see when you take a bat to him?*
PT: *He's curled up on the floor. I see it in the hall of my parent's house. He's hurt but he's not dead.*
TH: *How do you get him dead? How do you finish him off?*

PT: *Hit him until he's gone. Smash his head in with the bat.*
TH: *How does he look when you're done with him?*
PT: *I actually feel upset now (crying). He's my Dad.*
TH: *You wanted his love.*
PT: *He was good to me – but not good enough (sobbing).*
TH: *Just let yourself feel that searing grief.*
PT: *He gave me an awful life. He gave my mother an awful life. Even when I left the house, I had to take drugs to block out the pain.*

This was another very important moment. Not only had the patient finally allowed herself to feel her massive rage and searing grief, but she could experience deep compassion for herself, alleviating the need to punish herself.

TH: *Of course, there is so much pain that he caused.*
PT: *He couldn't understand my dyslexia. He's an academic and couldn't wrap his head around his child not being able to read. He would call me stupid and whack my fingers when I was trying to do my work. He took my head and smashed it against the sink.*
TH: *Oh my God.*
PT: *But yet I have feelings for him.*
TH: *It's so mixed. You loved him and wanted his love, but he was sadistic and that evokes this rage. So, to have rage toward someone you love, what does that evoke?*
PT: *I feel sick inside.*
TH: *That is a guilty feeling, huh? – to want to kill someone you love. So, you've been living with this terrible burden of guilt on top of the horrendous abuse. There is huge self-punishment in addition to all he inflicted on you – even choosing a man who would take over for him.*
PT: *All the men I chose were like that and I knew it! I thought I would be different than my Mom, and I would fight it, but I was worn down.*
TH: *That was your conscious mind, but now we see that unconsciously there was a need to be punished for the murderous rage you had toward your father. Have you done enough time?*
PT: *I think I have, yeah. I want out. I have even ruined my relationship to my children. They don't know me, and I don't really listen to them. I am so stressed I don't really listen. But, right now, I don't feel any of that tension. The turmoil in my stomach is gone. I feel calm and peaceful. Right how if my daughter came home and wanted to talk, I could just listen.*
TH: *That's really important to recognize. Now that you have let yourself feel these feelings instead of tensing up, keeping it inside and turning it on yourself, you feel peaceful and present. Then you could have caring relationships.*

In the follow-up to our initial session, the patient began by reflecting on the fact that she had never let herself cry over the deep pain she had experienced as a child. Our work together had helped her develop compassion for herself. This attitude seemed to extend, quite naturally, to forging a deeper connection with her children. She mentioned that all her typical anxiety and tension had disappeared after the session, allowing her to be present and relaxed with her children. She was able to listen to them and empathize with them, as she had with herself. Furthermore, she decided to pursue family therapy so that they could all share their feelings about everything that had happened, in a safe and neutral space.

To end this repetitive pattern of abuse in her relationships with men, the patient had to discover the internal forces responsible for it. Facing her mixed feelings toward her husband and father and coming to understand the role of guilt in perpetuating her suffering were essential steps in the process. Further work on the identification with her mother would be required. She was aware that she had identified with her mother rather than facing her feelings toward her – something she knew would be far more difficult than experiencing her true feelings toward her husband and father.

Summary

Working through unresolved emotional conflicts from the past, such that they are no longer repeated, but replaced with something healthy, is the ultimate goal of psychotherapy. This often requires many types and levels of intervention, depending on the forces responsible for the patient's symptoms, her level of ego adaptive capacity, and her ability to respond to intervention. Ultimately, it is the unconscious alliance, akin to an emotional immune system, that must overcome the forces of defenses and resistance to promote healing. The therapist is a facilitator of this process, but not the healing force itself. That force lies within, no matter how long it has been dormant. As Albert Schweitzer noted, "In everyone's life, at some time, an inner fire goes out. It is then burst into flame by an encounter with another human being." We should all be thankful for those people who rekindle that inner spirit.

Chapter 5

The Corrective Emotional Experience

Rupture and Repair

A Woman Abused – Follow-Up to the Trial Therapy

TH: *Why don't you start by telling me about the thoughts, feelings, and reactions to our first meeting?*

PT: *One thing I must say is that I have never been upset about what happened to me as a child with my father. What I mean is that I have never cried before, not as an adult and I'm not even sure I cried as a child. Usually, I just get angry and frustrated.*

TH: *Of course you were angry – that's a response to the unbelievable pain about being treated in such a brutal and sadistic fashion by the father you loved. It was as you said, "but it wasn't enough," that was when the pain broke through and you really felt that grief.*

PT: *I never felt that before. The other thing was that I had such unbearable pain about losing the baby, but at every anniversary I don't cry, I get angry, storm around and get into fights with everybody.*

TH: *So, what was it like to let yourself feel that pain and heartbreak – to get through that tough shield? You had been so guarded and hadn't let yourself be vulnerable.*

PT: *When I have been vulnerable in the past, I never got the right response. With my husband, I knew he didn't do crying – he never comforted me. My Dad was the same.*

TH: *There was no comfort there. So, when you felt that searing pain and the absolutely murderous rage toward both your husband and father, we also discovered guilt and saw how you were punishing yourself.*

PT: *Then I felt this amazing calm. All that awful anxiety that is always chewing up my stomach was gone. It was amazing. I needed that. Then I was able to be more present with my children. You know what's so interesting? It was only after you pointed the things I do to avoid – like looking away and how I laughed to cover up my feelings, that I realized it.*

DOI: 10.4324/9781003197669-5

After that session, my daughter told me something that upset her. She said, "Why are you laughing at me – why are you doing that? It's not funny." Maybe they have said it before, but I just never heard it, but this week I realized I was doing it again. This time I heard it and even thanked her for telling me. This time I heard her – I heard her because you had pointed it out. I do that!

TH: *It seems the session had quite an impact. What was different this time?*

PT: *This is the most I've ever got out of therapy by far – just from those few hours. I think because you pushed me. Before, when I would go quiet and avoided, they just moved back and there were long periods of silences. It was so awkward. I noticed you pushing me and being with me made so much difference. All that chaos I was living with inside is from the past. We were able to get to some of it so I could feel calm and clear in my head.*

TH: *Even though it was difficult to face what you had been avoiding, all that stress and anxiety, which is created by holding it all in, went away. I am sure there is more there, but it's a good start.*

Not only were the patient's parents emotionally unavailable, but previous therapists simply sat in silence and did not help the patient moderate anxiety or turn on defenses so that she could experience her true feelings. In contrast, she made it clear that calling attention to her defenses, while challenging her to face her true feelings, created an internal corrective experience, as well as an interpersonal one. By facing and experiencing emotions she had avoided all her life, she got into more intimate contact with her true self. Doing so enabled her to be a calm and responsive presence with her children. This kind of corrective emotional experience bolsters the alliance and speeds the process of change.

History of the Concept

Perhaps our patients are not the only ones who suffer from the repetition compulsion and the return of the repressed. Practitioners in our field seem to discover, forget, and then remember once again how vital the role of emotional experiencing is in the process of change. The patient recounted here made it clear that helping her experience feelings she had been avoiding – and being with her through it all – made all the difference. This constituted a corrective emotional experience, not only vis-à-vis her parents and husband, but previous therapists as well.

Initially, Bruer and Freud (1985/1995) focused on emotional abreaction as a vehicle for healing. Freud's early work was designed to unearth previously repressed id impulses by bypassing the ego and its defenses (with hypnosis, for example). While providing temporary relief, he discovered the phenomenon of the "return of the repressed" following catharsis, and concluded that the ego must be strengthened in order to tolerate and integrate unconscious feelings, wishes, and impulses into consciousness. Eventually, the analytic process became far too cognitive and intellectual, with an almost exclusive focus on the use of interpretation.

Ferenczi (1980) was one of the first to emphasize the importance of emotional involvement over intellectual insight in the therapeutic process. He advocated the expression of warmth, care, and concern on the therapist's part, rather than the "neutral" stance that was typical at the time. Doing so involved an attempt at creating a contrast to what he had assumed was a forbidding relationship with parents; an early precursor to the concept of the corrective emotional experience elucidated by Alexander and French (1946). Their groundbreaking research into the effectiveness of dynamic psychotherapy concluded that "only the actual experience of a new solution, in the transference or the patient's current life, gives him the conviction that a new solution is possible and induces him to give up the old neurotic pattern" (Alexander & French, 1946, p. 338). This is the essence of the "corrective emotional experience," which they concluded was the secret of every penetrating therapeutic result. To facilitate such an experience, the therapist must be conscious, intentional, and specific, in order to assure that he is providing an experience that is contradictory to that which is expected, rather than a repetition of troubled and dysfunctional relationship patterns established in the past.

In analytic circles, the tendency has been to stress the repetition of the old conflict in the transference relationship, emphasizing the *similarity* between the two. In contrast, the therapeutic significance of the *differences* in these relationships was often overlooked. Alexander and French (1946) discovered that it was just such a difference that provided therapeutic value. They contended that this very difference afforded the patient an opportunity to face again, *under more favorable circumstances*, emotions which were previously experienced as unbearable or unacceptable.

In addition to their focus on the corrective emotional experience, Alexander and French (1946) abandoned the analytic attitude of free-floating attention that was prevalent at the time. Instead, they stressed the value of "designing a plan of treatment based on a dynamic-diagnostic appraisal of the patient's personality and the actual problems he has to solve in his given life conditions" (p. 5). Their research concluded that insight was the *result*, rather than the *cause*, of therapeutic progress. They felt that the therapeutic process must include interventions designed to help patients: (1) abandon defenses; (2) directly experience and express anxiety-provoking feelings; (3) develop insight into their emotional conflicts, (4) assimilate the unconscious memories associated with those conflicts; and (5) above all, be provided "the corrective emotional experiences necessary to break up the old reaction pattern" (p. 26). They viewed the therapist as a facilitator rather than a healer. "Just as the healing of a wound is a natural function of the human body, so the integration of new insights is a normal function of the ego" (p. 27).

That said, skill and flexibility on the part of the therapist were considered essential in facilitating such an experience for each patient.

Many others have confirmed these early findings. Frieda Fromm Reichman declared that the patient is in need of an experience, not an explanation. Arieti (1974) emphasized the importance of providing a relational experience that had not been available to the patient with previous attachment figures. He suggested that this new type of experience was both a prerequisite for therapeutic success and a force for change in its own right.

It is important to note that most of these clinicians were adamant about the fact that it is not possible to "re-parent" the patient, or in any way directly make up for what he missed in childhood. Instead, by providing what Winnicott (1962) would have called a "facilitating environment" of empathy and attunement, the patient is helped to face the reality of her life, as well as her true feelings about it. Similarly, Malan (1976) stressed that undoing the past is not possible. The therapist is "corrective" in the sense that he is willing to face all the failures and losses the patient has incurred, in order to help him bear his feelings about them (including those experienced with the therapist himself).

Malan worked with Balint (1968), who emphasized the importance of making the patient a "counteroffer." In other words, the therapist must offer the patient a relationship that differs from his expectations. He found that this surprise offer tended to evoke deep feelings and promoted rapid change. This is very much in alignment with Freud's observation that "we feel in the contrast, not in the state of things."

Gill (1983, 1994) and Hoffman (1983) have also underscored the importance of offering the patient a new emotional experience, which included the direct examination of feelings evoked in the transference. The freedom to experience the kinds of feelings and perceptions patients have always avoided is corrective in and of itself. Secondarily, expressing and sharing these previously hidden feelings and wishes to the therapist is another opportunity for a contradictory and corrective relational experience. To facilitate such a process, it is essential that the therapist behave in ways that are distinctly different from early figures. In addition to providing a corrective experience, the explicit processing of the feelings evoked in these interactions is viewed as crucial in consolidating the process of change (Fosha, 2000). This processing must include feelings that are similar to those from the past, as well as the new and contradictory feelings evoked by the very different ways in which the therapist responds to the patient's daring self-expression.

Weiss and his colleagues (Silberschatz, 2005; Weiss, 1993) have suggested that our patients are highly motivated, albeit unconsciously, to test out their dysfunctional beliefs with the therapist, in the hopes that they will be refuted. In other words, they assert that patients generally come into therapy wanting to get better and hoping for a corrective emotional experience with the therapist. Good psychotherapy is a place where that can, and reliably does, happen. Unfortunately, there are also scenarios in which the pathological patterns of the past are repeated within the therapist-patient dyad. In these cases, patients drop out or get worse (as in the case of the Errant Priest, whose treatment was reviewed in this volume).

While Davanloo rarely, if ever, used the term "corrective emotional experience" when referring to his own work, those who observed it often did. In the late 1970s, there were two large international symposia on short-term dynamic psychotherapy, featuring Malan, Mann, Sifneos, and Davanloo, among others. Two books of the proceedings were subsequently published (Davanloo, 1978, 1980). Following almost every one of Davanloo's case presentations, the panelists commented on the centrality of the corrective emotional experience that he was able to foster with patients. This primarily involved his steady presence in encouraging an open and honest look at the patients' true feelings toward figures in his past and present life, as well as those stimulated in the transference.

After observing Davanloo's work via videotape, Marmor (1978) wrote an article in which he "revised" the notion of a corrective emotional experience. While Alexander and French (1946) were criticized for manipulating the transference, Marmor suggested that this was a gross misunderstanding of the concept. Instead, he observed that therapy is most likely to be corrective when the therapist responds in a considered fashion, based upon a precise and thorough psychodynamic understanding of the factors contributing to the development and maintenance of the patient's neurosis. The more precisely the therapist understands the patient's dynamics, the more likely he will be able to recognize the reactivation of the old conflict in the transference situation and be in a position to facilitate a new and corrective response (instead of repeating the old, destructive pattern). To reiterate, rather than emphasizing the *similarity* of the transference to past relationships or engaging in a re-enactment of past dysfunctional patterns, the therapist focused on responding *differently*. This often involves helping the patient face emerging feelings toward the therapist in an honest and direct manner, lest the defenses against such feelings distort the therapeutic relationship. Other models, such as Accelerated Empathic Dynamic Psychotherapy (Fosha, 2000), have emphasized the role of an empathic and emotionally corrective therapist as the main ingredient of transformation in the method. This stance is not without controversy (Ecker et al., 2012).

Another criticism of any attempt to supply a corrective emotional experience to the patient involved the abandonment of therapeutic neutrality. Alexander (Marmor, 1978) emphasized the fact that complete neutrality is neither possible nor desirable. Similarly, Davanloo eschewed the notion of therapeutic neutrality and urged therapists to take a stand for health and healing, suggesting this can only take place within an atmosphere of unsparing honesty. He did not value neutrality nor did he advise therapists to simply interpret the patient's behavior. Instead, he suggested they would need to apply pressure on patients to experience and express their true feelings toward others (including the therapist), as well as challenge their defenses against them. This is, in and of itself, a corrective experience, as few of us were ever invited to be emotionally honest with attachment figures.

Marmor (1978) also made a point of emphasizing that a corrective emotional experience must involve non-verbal, as well as verbal modes of communication; making special reference to Davanloo's direct eye contact and other invitations to emotional closeness. This point cannot be emphasized strongly enough. A therapist can say all the right things, but if his non-verbal behavior is contrary to the content of his message, it will not elicit a therapeutic response. When trainees are first learning, they are often very anxious about inviting feelings toward themselves in the transference. While they might say, "How do you experience this feeling toward me?", they do so in a very tentative fashion, with a quiet tone and a question mark in their voice, as if to say, "but let's not." In fact, tone of voice was considered very important to Davanloo (personal communication, 1988–1991), who encouraged trainees to maintain a tone of voice consistent with the affect or defense in question. If we are confronting a patient's self-destructive defenses, our tone will be firm and straightforward – calling a spade a spade and refusing to downplay or minimize the destructiveness of the ways in which the patient is treating himself. When we are inviting anger, our speech will likely be strong and clipped. In contrast, when grief emerges, our tone will be soft and soothing. In this way, Davanloo was an early advocate for the use of affective "mirroring," in which therapists seek to reflect the patient's underlying affect, all in an attempt to emotionally connect with the patient and facilitate healing.

In fact, it could be argued that Davanloo's (1990, 2000) method has been specifically designed to address and remove transference distortions so that the real relationship with the therapist can prevail. It is essential to remember that transference phenomena are a manifestation of defensive processes. The patient is seeing you, the therapist, not as you, but as someone from the past. Rather than interpret this to the patient, or try to talk him out of his distorted view, Davanloo (1990) welcomed the feelings activated in the transference. In fact, Davanloo (1990, 2000) discovered that an early focus on transference feelings was the key to the unlocking of the unconscious and paving the way to deep and rapid change. This early work on feelings toward the therapist was also intended to prevent the development of transference neurosis, which all too often hampers treatment efforts and can prove intractable (Freud, 1937).

By recognizing the emergence of the patient's core conflict in the transference as soon as possible, and inviting the patient to experience and express his anxiety-laden feelings and impulses openly (albeit in fantasy), the patient discovers who the therapist has come to represent. A transfer of images, in which the therapist's face and/or body are suddenly replaced by a figure from the past, is a cardinal sign of what Davanloo referred to as a "major unlocking of the unconscious." Once the patient has experienced the de-repression of previously avoided feelings and memories regarding primary attachment figures, the need to defend against them via transference distortion is no longer necessary. The therapist becomes who she is – a helpful collaborator – rather than a stand-in for someone else. This allows for new and corrective experiences going forward, instead of a re-enactment of outmoded and destructive patterns in relationships.

While there are times when one intense and corrective experience with the therapist is all that is required to remediate the defense of displacement and transference, in other cases this process needs to be repeated multiple times throughout the course of treatment. For example, a paternal transference might need to be worked through multiple times – each time the transference phenomenon reflects a different facet of the paternal relationship or a different set of feelings toward the same figure. Alternatively, the therapist can come to represent different figures at different times – from parents to grandparents and siblings. All such feelings, impulses, and fantasies need to be addressed in a direct and straightforward manner in order to work through, integrate, and resolve them.

Following each breakdown of defenses and subsequent breakthrough of previously avoided feelings toward the therapist, the patient is helped to see more clearly how he has distorted the present through the filter of the past, both with the therapist and others in his current life. Once the links between past and present are made, the patient is able to distinguish between these figures to an ever-greater degree.

Alterations in One's Sense of Self

So far, we have focused on the importance of facilitating a corrective emotional experience in the interpersonal realm. In addition to this, it is often necessary to promote a corrective emotional experience within the patient himself. What does this mean?

We have reviewed the understanding of the corrective emotional experience from analytic and dynamic perspectives; yet even cognitive behavior therapists like David Barlow (2000, Barlow et al., 2011) have come to appreciate the central role that emotional awareness, regulation, and expression have on the therapeutic process (as well as a healthy life). Since deficits in emotional awareness and regulation are a foundational aspect of all psychiatric disorders, Barlow (2000) advised a shift in therapeutic focus from conscious cognitions to the internal emotional life of the patient. While he has not specifically addressed the concept of the corrective emotional experience in his writing (to my knowledge), he does suggest the necessity of exposing patients to the thoughts, feelings, and wishes he has been too anxious to acknowledge and reveal in the past. Doing so often provides a corrective experience as the patient discovers, in an experiential manner, that they are not dangerous at all.

In fact, when patients freely experience emotions they have long been repressing, it is often with surprise and delight that they discover how enlivening they are. In this way, the patient is having an *internal* corrective emotional experience. Furthermore, allowing and embracing all his feelings is an experience of authenticity and spontaneity that often proves profoundly life-affirming. This is an internal experience and does not necessarily require an interpersonal component. Ecker et al. (2012) seem especially strident on this point, asserting that it is the patient's discovery of his own inner life, no longer obscured by limiting beliefs, that is essential for a corrective adjustment. That said, Ecker is a highly attuned, empathic, and facilitating presence – a factor that can't be discounted or ignored in the success of his interventions.

Wolstein (1985, 1987) and Fiscalini (1990) have also underscored the ameliorative effect of a new experience of self, rather than just that of the other. It is the relationship of a new, stronger, more whole, and powerful self that is truly life-altering in their view. Wolstein (1985) asserted that deep change is the consequence of the patient having lived through (not simply worked through) his anxiety, pain, and rage long enough and deeply enough to encounter his "true self." This kind of new experience of self, in the here and now, revealed without masks, diversions, and defenses, is profoundly corrective and therapeutic. "Changes in self-organization take place as the patient recovers and experiences fully hidden or disclaimed aspects of the self" (Kavanaugh, 1985). Diana Fosha (2000) has also emphasized the therapeutic effects of experiencing the self as whole and healthy. In fact, most of her clinical innovations have been in the area of processing the sense of the self as "new," "healed," "whole," and "transformed" following the experience of change.

Ultimately, the essence of the corrective emotional experience involves re-exposing the patient, "under favorable circumstances, to emotional situations which he could not handle in the past" (Alexander & French, 1946, p. 66). The "difference between the new feelings and the old have sometimes been overlooked and the importance of these differences many times underestimated" according to Alexander and French (1946). Many therapists focus exclusively on problems and conflicts, prioritizing the past, while neglecting the new and corrective experience of current relationships, including that with a therapist. That said, it has been suggested (Alexander & French, 1946; Fosha, 2000) that simply providing a new experience is insufficient to produce therapeutic change. First of all, the patient must be present and engaged, so that he is open to that new experience. Then, the feelings triggered by this new and corrective experience must be experienced and expressed. The contrast between this new experience and the typical pattern, established in the past and repeated throughout his life, must be made conscious and explicit in order to interrupt old neurotic patterns and create new alternatives.

Clinical Examples

Unintentional Corrective Experiences

Sometimes a corrective emotional experience is required *before* the patient can open up, develop trust, and engage at a deep level; while at other times, this only happens once the patient has taken the risk to do so. The following two examples were spontaneous responses by the therapist, rather than those consciously and intentionally employed in the hopes of providing a corrective experience. However, in both cases, new and corrective experiences with the therapist created an opening, allowing a close and trusting relationship to develop.

Long before cell phones were ubiquitous, a highly intelligent and professionally accomplished patient, who used her verbal acumen and tendency toward self-sufficiency to create an impenetrable barrier to emotional closeness, was seen for a trial therapy. Early efforts to acquaint her with these defenses and their attendant cost (including distance from me and inevitable therapeutic failure) were largely unsuccessful. Despite a relative lack of progress in the initial session, the patient seemed eager to return for a follow-up appointment.

During our first session, the patient mentioned having arranged for a cab to pick her up and take her to the airport for a flight back home. After finishing up at the office, I walked to my car, only to see her standing in the distance, waiting for the taxi that should have arrived a half hour earlier. I approached her and asked what had happened. She told me that the cab never showed up. She was in danger of missing her flight. Since the airport was only five miles from my office, I told her to get in the car so I could take her there myself. She initially declined the offer, not wanting to put me out, but I assured her it would be no trouble at all. In fact, I let her know it would be a pleasure to help her out. We rode quietly to the airport, and she thanked me when I dropped her off at the terminal. In the following session, she revealed having been deeply touched by my actions and experienced my sincere and spontaneous expression of care in a way that words alone had not.

While I had not consciously thought of this as a therapeutic strategy, and was simply responding as one human being to another, I came to realize that my response stood in stark contrast to what she had experienced in her family of origin. From the earliest time, she had been encouraged to need nothing and no one, and to take care of herself as well as others. She became tearful as she expressed her gratitude toward me and contrasted this new experience with so many she had had in her life. She had gotten used to being on her own and was terrified of depending on anyone. This spontaneous gesture on my part had a marked effect on her view of me and of what was possible in a relationship. Therapy began in earnest.

A male patient in his mid-40s came for help with debilitating anxiety and depression that had resulted in several hospitalizations and therapies over the previous 25 years, none of which had been very helpful. He had been raised by a sadistic, demanding father, and a cold, detached mother. There was no room for feelings and emotions in the family – only for actions and achievements. He had gone to the most prestigious schools in the country, but after graduation from college fell into a serious depression, resulting in his first hospitalization. Unfortunately, most of his previous therapeutic experiences were not at all ameliorative. In fact, they only reinforced his sense of being misunderstood, and fortified his belief that he would never get his needs met in a relationship. As a result, his tough-guy façade and cold detachment only increased over time and were difficult, if not impossible, to penetrate.

Then, one day, he passed me in the hallway on my way to the rest room. I was crying; having just received some very bad news. He was rarely early for sessions, and I never imagined I would bump into him, but that's just what happened. After pulling myself together and asking him to come into my consulting room, I was shocked by the sudden and dramatic shift in his demeanor. He sat forward and asked me how I was. I replied that I had received some sad news but was fine and ready to work. He went on to tell me about the profound effect that seeing me crying had on him. Prior to this, he had perceived my professional manner as a replica of his mother's cold, icy detachment. The pressure I put on him to abandon defenses was experienced as something akin to the taunting his father confronted him with on daily basis. Given these transferential perceptions, he was damned if he was going to reveal himself to me. Suddenly, he saw me as a caring and sensitive woman, and he opened up in response. Once again, this seemingly random event created an opening for a new relationship that, in each case, proved highly therapeutic. Such things cannot be manufactured or manipulated and must be sincere. However, they must be examined thoroughly, and the feelings evoked in the encounter processed explicitly. In other words, it is not sufficient to simply behave differently from early attachment figures, but to facilitate the direct experience of the feelings evoked by such a contrast.

Intentional Corrective Experiences Prior to the Breakthrough

In many cases, a good deal of therapeutic work must be accomplished before the patient is prepared for, or receptive to, a corrective experience. In contrast to the two examples already given, in most cases, these experiences are intentionally facilitated by the therapist. To accomplish this end, the patient must become acquainted with the defenses he uses to create a resistance to closeness with the therapist, so he can choose to relinquish them. In some patients, this clears the path to a genuine experience of feelings and creates the opportunity for a new and corrective emotional experience. In other cases, the process of acquainting the patient with their defenses is far more demanding and time consuming.

It should also be noted that being encouraged to face and experience rage directly toward the therapist is often highly corrective. It is extremely rare for attachment figures to welcome anger. In fact, it is typically prohibited and punished. Not only do no feared negative consequences ensue following such a therapeutic encounter, but feelings of closeness and deep understanding typically follow.

Corrective Experiences after a Breakthrough

Alterations in one's sense of self, from damaged to whole and from false/fractured to authentic/integrated, are essential for long-term change. However, research suggests that only those who get emotionally involved in the process achieve this outcome (Pennebaker, 1997). Insights must be consolidated following the breakthrough of feeling and de-repression of memories shedding light on core conflicts. Profound corrective emotional experiences, in which the patient experiences herself and her relationships with others from a new vantage point, most often take place *after* the breakdown of defenses and breakthrough of previously avoided feelings. This often leads to a revised and more nuanced sense of self.

The Fee Increase

A male patient in his mid-30s had developed an entrenched pattern of passivity, compliance, and subservience, which inevitably resulted in feelings of helplessness and depression. He focused on the needs, feelings, and wishes of others while failing to consider his own. In the mid-phase of treatment, I raised my rates. I alerted him to this change in an email, suggesting we discuss it in our next session.

PT: *I got your message about the fee increase (looking anxious and avoiding my eyes).*

TH: *What kinds of feelings and reactions are you having?*

PT: *Of course, I understand and it's your right to increase the fee, but I'm really upset.*

TH: *What do you mean by upset? What is the feeling toward me for raising the fee in the midst of your treatment?*

PT: *I understand but it's really tough for me. I don't have insurance and pay out of pocket (getting a bit weepy).*

TH: *Let's look at this, because it seems to me we are seeing a very familiar pattern here. I ask how you feel toward me and you tell me what you think or what you do, while your feelings are omitted.*

PT: *Well I'm sad – what if I can't pay? Am I taking too long? Maybe I should have been done by now and this is your way of kicking me in the pants to get going.*

TH: *Do you see how you avoid declaring the feeling toward me? It goes back on you instead. As if you are the problem. I am the one changing the agreement.*

It is essential that the therapist acknowledge her role in the interaction in question. The fact is, the therapist had raised her rates. Rather than indulge in justification for so doing, an examination of the patient's feelings and characteristic manner of responding was the most pressing and immediate therapeutic task.

PT: *That's true – I do that. It's never the other person – always me in the wrong.*

TH: *So is that what you want to do here or do you want to face the feelings toward me?*

PT: *Now that you mention is, I didn't like the way you presented it in an email and, frankly, I think it's too much of an increase all at once.*

TH: *Let's discuss it – that's important, but I am still wondering about the feeling toward me.*

PT: *I realize now that I'm angry about it (still a bit weepy).*

TH: *Great. How do you experience that? Let's see if you can feel the anger without covering it over with tears.*

PT: *Yeah, I am sick of that. I do feel it. It's actually sharper now and I am more energized. It's a little anxiety provoking but I am also feeling touched that you said we can discuss it.*

TH: *Of course. There are two of us in this relationship.*

In this case, a number of conflicts were involved. The patient had an intrapsychic conflict regarding anger toward loved ones. Additionally, he had a pattern of avoiding interpersonal conflict by ignoring his own needs and feelings and complying with the real or imagined demands of the other. This constituted what Stan Tatkin (2012) has referred to as a one-person system. To highlight this distortion and provide a corrective experience, it was not enough simply to focus on the patient's mixed feelings toward the therapist. In addition, it was imperative to suggest the possibility that there would be room for two in our relationship.

PT: *In a strange way that never occurred to me.*

TH: *Your tendency is to only consider one person in the relationship – usually the other – and then to accommodate to their wishes. How is that working?*

PT: *Not well, but, yeah, it's been "like it or lump it".*
TH: *So, how about if we do it differently and consider your needs and feelings as well as mine?*

Rather than simply focus on the cost of the patients' defensive mode of operation, presenting a clear and healthy alternative, while putting the patient at choice, paved the way for the possibility of a corrective experience.

PT: *Yeah, that's great. I would want to say...*
TH: *Want to or will?*
PT: *I will. I am going to use that anger to assert myself and ask if we can split the difference and have a smaller increase.*
TH: *That sounds fair.*
PT: *Really? This is great. I never imagined this and thought, "that's just the way it is". She is raising the fee and there is nothing I can do about it. I can suck it up and pay or stop therapy. Yeah, now I realize I was really mad and thinking, "She's unfair. I don't like the way she did this."*
TH: *And if I hadn't brought it up and encouraged you to declare you wishes and feelings, or to choose a new, what would have happened?*
PT: *It wouldn't have been good for me or the relationship. This is always what happens. I suck it up and accommodate to keep the peace but then end up resentful and feeling as if I'm getting taken advantage of.*
TH: *How does it feel to consider your own needs and feelings here and to speak up in your own behalf?*
PT: *It feels great actually. I also feel closer to you. If I kept this to myself, I would have started to feel resentful and go to that helpless, victim place. It feels good to turn that around.*

In this session, a corrective emotional experience was facilitated following a disruption in the relationship. The therapist had announced an increase in the fee, which clearly evoked feelings in the patient that he was avoiding in his characteristic but ultimately self-defeating manner. He was passively accepting the announcement as a dictate, while burying his true feelings toward the therapist. Gone unattended, this process would likely result in a festering resentment that would undermine the connection. Instead of repeating this destructive pattern, the patient was alerted to its presence in our interaction and given the choice to repeat a self-defeating manner of relating, or to choose a new, more constructive path. With encouragement, the patient chose to face his feelings honestly and speak up on his own behalf. Doing so prevented a repetition of an unhealthy pattern while promoting a corrective experience.

Material obtained in the following session confirmed the therapeutic impact this experience had on the patient. Emboldened by his experience with the therapist, he was motivated to turn on the defenses of suppression and compliance and consider his own relational needs. These changes were translated into his life outside of the consulting room. He proudly reported having spoken up in a forthright manner to a number of authority figures to whom he would have deferred to in the past. Furthermore, he did so without anxiety and with an increasing sense of mastery and confidence.

The Woman Who Thought She Was a Bad Mother

A middle-aged married mother of two teenage boys came for help with life-long anxiety and depression, accompanied by a highly judgmental and critical internal voice, laced with perfectionistic demands. Since becoming a mother, the focus of this running commentary was largely about her being a bad and inadequate mother. She had been in therapy since adolescence and has been on SSRIs for over 20 years. Our initial work involved uncovering suppressed feelings of rage and guilt toward parents, as well as jealousy of siblings and childhood friends, which had been acted out in destructive ways during adolescence and prompting her to conclude that she was "a psychopath."

Our early work together had a marked impact in reducing the patient's symptoms and motivated her to go off medication. Consequently, she could feel herself come back to life, as the fog of antidepressants lifted, and the energy of her true feelings and desires was untethered. She realized how the numbness created by these drugs had increased her characterological passivity, allowing life to simply happen to her.

Once she could freely experience her own feelings and desires, a sense of personal agency re-emerged, enabling her to go after and create what she most wanted. She became particularly aware of feelings in her body that had been anesthetized for decades. She had been conflicted about her body, as she developed very large breasts at an early age, attracting unwanted attention from boys and men. This was internalized and turned against herself prior to therapy. As she faced her feelings toward others, she could accept all of herself – her physical body, as well as her feelings and desires. These corrective experiences took place after the breakthrough of previously repressed feelings toward others.

PT: *I noticed immediate and amazing changes after our last session. I walked upstairs and had a completely new kind of experience with my son* (who has been very difficult in the past). *Then, on Saturday night, after making love with my husband I felt so peaceful and thought, "There is light and dark inside me and that's OK".*

TH: *This sounds really important. Let's start with the first one and tell me how you felt inside.*

PT: *I felt good inside. When I went to see Jack* (her son), *I felt clear. I had no agenda and was able to be fully present with him. Usually I have and agenda, like "get off your iPad" – always trying to control him.*

TH: *Sounds like you are saying "When I get anxious, I get controlling". It's as if you're trying to control externals so you don't have to feel uncomfortable feelings inside. In contrast, when you are calm, you can be present. What allowed you to be in that space?*

PT: *I think it was experiencing that rage toward my sister and some others from the past and realizing how that was getting triggered by my son. In the past, it was as if I wasn't capable of handling my feelings or the situation – as if I was that scared, angry kid again. Now I am me, in the present, and I can deal with it calmly. Amazing.*

As in other cases described in this volume, the patient was having a dramatically corrective view of self which was immediately translated into new and corrective patterns of interaction with others. The change, in this case, took place from the inside out.

TH: *It also seemed to me – and I'm really interested on your take on this – that it was really important in the last session that you "got" that what you DO when you are anxious is not who you ARE. You had thought, "That must be the way I am. I must be a psychopath."*

PT: *Yes.*

TH: *Both the experience of those previously forbidden feelings and the deep understanding of yourself seemed equally important.*

PT: *Yes, and there was another big change I noticed. On Saturday night I made love with my husband. Usually, afterward, I have a hard time falling asleep. I will either ruminate and worry or think about my parenting. This time, I thought, "I have light and dark inside. I don't have to deny the dark." I felt completely whole and peaceful – being both, instead of trying to change the darkness or deny it.*

TH: *By darkness you mean?*

PT: *Anger, jealousy, or any feeling I had considered bad.*

TH: *That's a big turnaround. What would you say was responsible for the changes you describe?*

PT: *Our work together.*

TH: *Could you be more specific?*

PT: *What you mentioned – the difference between what I have done and who I am. That is very freeing. It's Ok to have all these feelings. It's not the same as acting on them, as I tended to do as a teenager. It was also working on the issues around closeness. My husband and I used to smoke pot before making love. That was also because I was on those SSRIs, which killed my sexual feelings. Now I am in my body, can feel my desire, and my love for him. I asked that we not use pot so we could be fully present with one another. It was great.*

It is best to assess, rather than assume, we understand the nature of the conflicts responsible for a patient's suffering. The therapeutic task involves a process of unearthing *all* the anxiety-provoking and guilt-laden feelings the patient has defensed against in ways that have created and perpetuated her suffering. Such feelings are typically very mixed and must be experienced and integrated into a coherent narrative in order to produce robust change. As this patient mentioned, the result of this emotionally intense work was a new experience of self as a whole, complex, and multifaceted.

As the patient relinquished defenses (and got off SSRIs), she was able to connect with her true feelings, wishes, and desires. Guilt about these feelings had been largely responsible for her need to suppress them, while simultaneously demanding an exclusive focus on the needs and wishes of others. As she was able to face, tolerate, and integrate her previously avoided feelings, her old pattern of subservience and compliance was replaced with healthy self-assertion. Furthermore, she was able to be fully present with both her husband and sons, allowing those relationships to blossom. The ability to shift and repair those relationships further bolstered her previously precarious self-esteem.

The Role of the Therapist

In examining the role of the corrective emotional experience in successful psychotherapy, it becomes clear that the therapist must resist becoming part of the problem, and needs to take an active role in being part of the solution. Many have emphasized the importance of the therapist's authenticity and spontaneity in facilitating such a process (Greenberg & Pinsof, 1986; Hoffman, 1987). How can we help patients reclaim and express their authentic selves if we are hiding behind a mask? Ehrenberg (2010) has referred to the authentic or real relationship between therapist and patient as existing on an "intimate edge." She has emphasized the importance of the therapist being actively and authentically engaged, rather than coolly detached. Only then can she, with a sense of integrity, confront detachment on the patient's part. Ehrenberg (2010) and Safran (Reading et al., 2019) have advocated a highly collaborative therapeutic relationship in which thoughts, feelings, needs, and desires are made explicit.

In sum, there is considerable agreement in the field that therapists must become highly skilled and specific in their interventions (given an understanding of the patient's specific dynamics) if they are going to be effective. Accordingly, no one size fits all approach, or standard intervention based upon a manual, will suffice in creating deep and lasting change in a consistent manner over time and across patients. Our specific case conceptualization must guide our interventions. For example, we would treat a patient who had been deprived of warmth and pressured to accomplish goals at any cost very differently from one who had been coddled and overly praised for the slightest effort.

In addition to responding differently than key figures from the past, we must calibrate our interventions in such a way as to reach the patient at his highest level of ego adaptive capacity. Recently, a colleague requested supervision on a new case. This middle-aged woman had been horrendously abused as a child and had repeated a pattern of allowing herself to be used and abused by men. Just before reaching out for help, she caught her husband rubbing himself up against their 17-year-old granddaughter. She allowed herself to feel the rage about this violation that she had never experienced regarding her own history of abuse. This crisis prompted her to seek treatment. The therapist was surprised to find that, despite her history, the patient proved highly motivated, responsive, and capable of facing strong conflicted feelings without undue anxiety. The therapist encouraged honesty and challenged the patient to face all the feelings of rage toward perpetrators that she had avoided all her life. This therapist's use of pressure and challenge was received as a refreshing vote of confidence in her ability to deal with life courageously. The results were rapid and significant. A similar dynamic was present in the case of "A Woman Abused" in this volume.

Summary

Understanding the nature and importance of facilitating a corrective emotional experience in psychotherapy, on both internal and interpersonal levels, has been the focus of this chapter. In some cases, a corrective emotional experience is required in order to overcome resistance and begin the therapeutic process, while in other cases, this experience transpires after defenses have broken down and feelings have broken through the repressive barrier. Examples of both such processes were included.

Chapter 6

Rupture and Repair

Introduction

Relationships are messy. Therapeutic relationships are no exception. When first learning Intensive Short-Term Dynamic Psychotherapy (ISTDP), I was so determined to be effective and efficient in my interventions, that I sometimes missed the forest for the trees – running over the patient in my zeal for a cure. A particularly painful example of this involved one of my first ISTDP cases: a middle-aged woman who embodied the stereotype of a schoolmarm, driven by rigid standards and deeply committed to doing right by her students, but isolated and inhibited in her personal life. She had never dated and had few friends; she was plagued by social anxiety and felt quite depressed. These symptoms were the focus of therapeutic intervention and, on that level, were successful. Her anxiety was dramatically reduced, and her depression lifted after 10–12 sessions. As soon as these goals were achieved, I suggested termination. The patient readily agreed, and the process proceeded smoothly, as had the treatment as a whole.

When contacted a year later to schedule a follow-up session (as is my practice), she responded by saying, "I couldn't possibly come back to see you." I was shocked by her comment and asked her to tell me more.

> I was utterly devastated when you suggested we end the therapy. I was feeling better *because* of our relationship. I finally found someone who seemed to care about me and my feelings. When you suggested we end therapy, I was beside myself.

"I am so sorry," I replied, "I had no idea. I'd like to offer you a session, free of charge, to come and talk about all this so we can sort it out." "Why would I talk with you about this?" she replied. "As soon as I got better, you got rid of me. I was foolish to think you actually cared about me. This is so upsetting to talk about, I just can't go there." With that, she said goodbye and hung up.

DOI: 10.4324/9781003197669-6

Now I was the one who felt devastated. How could I have so misread this woman? Why hadn't she spoken up when I suggested termination and, further, why wouldn't she accept my apology, along with the opportunity to talk it through and possibly make it right? These questions haunted me. Studying the science of relationships has shed light on this painful episode and helped me prevent such disasters going forward.

Infant research and data on positive outcomes in psychotherapy suggest that disruptions to our attachments are not a problem in and of itself. In fact, disruptions are the norm and seem to serve an essential function, promoting growth and resilience (Tronick & Gold, 2020). The decisive factor is how these disruptions are handled – whether they are ignored and denied or acknowledged and repaired. Just as with broken bones, relationships that break down and heal are stronger and more resilient than those that were never tested. Being able to acknowledge and repair misunderstandings increases trust. Failure to do so leads to breakdowns in communication and, in therapy, to premature termination and negative outcomes.

Stan Tatkin (2012), a noted couple's therapist, has suggested that "nothing is harder than another human being." When we fail to allow for the messiness and struggle of relationships, we do ourselves and others a disservice. Sue Johnson (2019), who developed Emotion Focused Therapy for Couples (EFT), has discovered that relationships are a constant process of connecting, missing, and misreading cues, disconnecting, repairing, and finding deeper connection as a result. It is like a dance of meeting and parting and finding each other again. Success in life and relationships is not about achieving perfection. Rather, healthy relationships require us to acknowledge mistakes, misunderstandings, and even the ruptures in relationships so that we can repair any damage done and rebuild trust. We don't know what we are made of or how strong our relationships are until they are tested. When everything is copacetic, it's easy to be kind and generous, but how do you behave when things don't go your way? It turns out that our ability to detect breakdowns in communication and to put them right is one of the most important factors in sustaining healthy relationships that we have discovered (Gottman & DeClaire, 2002; Tronick & Gold, 2020). This is as true for parents and children and teachers and students as it is for clinicians and surgeons (Gawande, 2004).

In this chapter, we will review the topic of rupture and repair in the therapeutic alliance, as well as examine the support for the notion that this process is ubiquitous in all human relations. We will discuss how to identify and repair these ruptures, whether large or small, intentional or accidental. The need to balance the development of safety in the therapeutic relationship with the necessity of challenge, often creating disruption, will be a central focus. In addition to clinical examples, we will include theoretical considerations and empirical results to the discussion.

Connection and Disconnection: Research Findings

The first step in the rupture-repair process involves the therapist's ability to *identify* the therapeutic blunders and missteps that lead to rupture and disconnection (Safran & Kraus, 2014). This is one area where experience seems to matter. Research suggests that experienced therapists are more accurate in their detection of therapeutic ruptures than their less experienced colleagues (Talbot et al., 2019). At the same time, other research (Binder & Strupp, 1997) reveals that therapists generally overestimate their ability to handle such breakdowns and conflicts adroitly. Anxious therapists proved less able to respond to patient identification of ruptures with empathy than their securely attached counterparts. Furthermore, therapists were more likely to respond well to disruption in the alliance with anxious and preoccupied patients than those who tend to be dismissive.

When comparing therapist and patient views of alliance ruptures, interesting differences emerge. Therapists in one study (Eames & Roth, 2000) detected ruptures to the alliance in over 50% of the sessions studied, while patients reported such disruptions in less than 20% of the sessions reviewed (Eames & Roth, 2000). That said, therapists tended to attribute the source of the rupture to the patient and often failed to see their own role in creating or perpetuating the misunderstanding (Safran & Kraus, 2014; Safran & Muran, 2000; Safran, Muran & Eubanks-Careter, 2011). This is a troubling finding, as other research (Coutinho, Ribeiro, HIll & Safran, 2011) has indicated that patients are quite hesitant to directly voice their disagreement or disappointment with the therapist and only do so when an invitation to examine the relationship is initiated by the clinician.

The lack of attention to ruptures, as well as the therapist's hesitance to acknowledge his own role in the breakdown of the alliance, may well be a major cause of premature dropouts in psychotherapy (Bordin, 1994). Sadly, despite reams of research on psychotherapy outcomes, and the development of hundreds of different treatment models, our ability to engage patients in treatment and prevent early withdrawal has not improved over the past 50 years. Outcome data suggest that approximately 35% of all patients seeking an initial consultation with a mental health professional fail to attend a second session, and 50% drop out by session 3 (Barrett et al., 2008). Since research indicates that at least 12 sessions are required for us to help 50% of our patients to recover (Hansen, Lambert & Forman, 2002), we have much room for improvement.

There is accumulating evidence (Safran & Krauss, 2014; Strauss et al., 2006) that therapeutic relationships in which there are episodes of rupture and repair are more impactful than those that run smoothly (or seem to, as the case discussed at the opening to this chapter illustrates). Therefore, being attuned to indications of misalignment, in order to correct course, is an essential skill to hone. Emerging research suggests that monitoring the alliance in real time, using observation, rather than a paper and pencil measure, has proved most effective (Coutinho et al., 2014; Safran & Kraus, 2014). That said, measures such as the OQ-45 have proven helpful in detecting dips in the alliance and patient regression, allowing therapists to reverse course and keep therapies on track (Beckstead et al., 2003).

Safran and colleagues (Safran & Kraus, 2014) have developed training courses specifically designed to help therapists assess the alliance over the course of treatment. Such training has emphasized the importance of maintaining an intensive focus on the here and now of the therapeutic relationship (with an emphasis on exploration of context). This step-by-step approach includes (1) detection of ruptures on the therapist's part (including non-verbal cues); (2) exploration of thoughts and feelings regarding the rupture; (3) encouraging the patient to overcome resistance to exploring his feelings regarding the rupture; (4) understanding the meaning of the misunderstanding; and (5) exploring what the patient needs and wishes in order to resolve the conflict (Safran et al., 2011). By encouraging "patients to explore, challenge, and change maladaptive interpersonal patterns" that contribute to ruptures, "the patient gradually develops more flexible and adaptive ways of negotiating interpersonal exchanges and learns that relationships are possible even when there is not always perfect accord" (Safran & Kraus, 2014, p. 382). In addition to this focused exploration in the here and now interaction between patient and therapist, an exploration of parallels and links to a pattern of disruptions in the patient's current and past relationships is important to include in the discussion. In the end, repaired alliance ruptures often constitute a corrective emotional experience.

Audiovisual recording of sessions is an invaluable tool in this process. By reviewing recorded sessions, we can observe what we did not detect – or had misinterpreted – during the session. Having an audiovisual record of the session to review (on our own and with colleagues and supervisors) can help us identify verbal and non-verbal signs that the patient is detaching, and the process is suffering. Noticing that the patient turns away from the therapist, avoiding eye contact, crossing his arms, or slowing down his rate of speech are all signs that something is amiss. Research suggests that therapists often miss such signs of hidden negative feelings coming up toward them (Hill et al., 1993). Detecting these negative responses and encouraging an open, honest, and direct expression of them is one of the key steps in the rupture-repair cycle. It is also important to conduct follow-up interviews to determine whether therapeutic efforts have had a lasting effect (Malan, 1979).

Our field has tended to focus almost exclusively on the therapist's intervention, rather than tracking the patient's *response* to intervention. The works of Strupp (Strupp & Hadley, 1979), Safran (Safran et al., 1990, 2011; Samstag, Muran & Safran, 2004), and Davanloo (1978, 1979, 1990, 2000) are notable exceptions. Their focus on the patient's emotional response to what the therapist offers has been a radical departure from models that focus on adherence to manuals and prescribed techniques. Clinician researchers such as Malan (1963, 1976, 1979; Malan & Coughlin Della Selva, 2007) have reminded us that developmental history and DSM diagnosis are poor prognostic indicators. Instead, response to intervention in the here and now has proven to provide the most timely and reliable source of information on the patient's ability to respond to treatment efforts.

Research from other fields is also pertinent here. Atul Gawande's research (2004) suggests that the best surgeons (those with the best outcomes) are not more technically skilled than their average colleagues. In fact, they make just as many mistakes as their less effective cohorts. However, the most effective surgeons track the patient's response to intervention assiduously and act quickly to change course when things do not proceed according to plan. They are masters at responding to failure and preventing a negative therapeutic response from becoming a catastrophe.

Similarly, Castonguay and his colleagues (1996) found that the most common cause of therapeutic misalliances is the therapist's rigidity in proceeding with their method, while ignoring the patient's response. When a strain in the alliance was detected, these therapists tended to view the patient as the problem and carried on with their intervention, even when there was no agreement or buy-in on the part of the patient (Binder & Strupp, 1997; Castonguay et al., 2010). In contrast, the most effective therapists demonstrated humility, with an ability to acknowledge errors and their own contribution to stalled or disrupted treatments. In addition, they make efforts to correct course. Furthermore, data suggest that growth and insight in both patient and therapist often result when therapists recognize a problem in the alliance and address it forthrightly (Safran & Muran, 2000). As Jung suggested, "The meeting of two personalities is like the contact of two chemical substances. If there is any reaction, both are transformed."

Repair Attempts

The type of repair attempt required depends upon the nature of the rupture. Is there a disagreement about the nature of the problem, the goals to be achieved, or the therapeutic task? Are these agreements in place but something is amiss at the level of the emotional bond? Aspland and colleagues (2008) found that disagreements about tasks and goals often go unspoken and can only be resolved once the therapist detects them and brings them into the conversation. Furthermore, they found that resolution to the disagreement only took place once the therapist shifted out of his own perspective and tried to understand the patient's experience. Once this understanding has been achieved, agreement about goals and tasks can be reestablished. To do so, it is rarely enough to acknowledge the rupture and apologize but, in order to be therapeutic, a repair must elicit the patient's thoughts and feelings about what has transpired (Safran

& Kraus, 2014). Furthermore, the patient's response to the therapist's repair attempt is very diagnostic. Does the patient attribute the disruption to themselves ("I guess I'm not very important."), to the therapist ("You seem rather scatterbrained and disorganized."), or to the relationship ("I think we just misunderstood one another.")? Do they accept the repair attempt and the invitation to explore the disruption or dismiss it with a comment like, "It's no big deal – no problem"? These responses contain a good deal of diagnostic information.

Gottman & DeClaire (2002) discovered that, in troubled relationships, repair attempts were often offered by one partner, but ignored or rejected out of hand by the other. In fact, response to repair attempts seemed to be the decisive factor in supporting the health and longevity of relationships. The same could be said of therapeutic relationships. Research indicates that dismissive responses are most likely to go unheeded (Rubino et al., 2010) and require tenacity on the part of the therapist. If the therapist allows himself to be dismissed, the opportunity to repair the disruption will be lost, and the alliance will suffer. Even when "small," these unacknowledged missteps tend to accumulate and lead to more serious deterioration over time. As Gottman (Gottman & DeClaire, 2002) has suggested more die of 10,000 papercuts than a knife in the back. In fact, flagrant ruptures in marriage, such as affairs or financial infidelity, are most likely to occur in the context of relationships in which small ruptures went chronically unattended. In all likelihood, a similar phenomenon can be detected in therapeutic relationships that go awry. The example given at the opening of this chapter is an example of both an unintentional disruption to the alliance and a case in which repair attempts were dismissed and refused.

Intentional Disruption

Healthy relationships achieve a balance between safety and challenge, whether they involve a parent and child, teacher and student, or therapist and patient dyad. It has been suggested that therapists, teachers, and parents have made the mistake of focusing excessively on safety, while failing to include sufficient challenge in their relationships (Tronick & Gold, 2020). The results have been catastrophic. Levels of anxiety, depression, and suicide among children and teens have reached a level two and three times that of generations past (Lukinoff & Haidt, 2019). Could it be that having been over protected and sheltered from life, we have failed to help this generation develop the resilience required to bounce back from adversity? This tendency can be reinforced in the therapeutic relationship when therapists rely too heavily on support and safety, rather than creating an environment in which challenge to the status quo, taking risks, and tolerating anxiety for growth is encouraged (Schnarch, 1991).

Winnicott (1963) was likely the first analyst to emphasize the need for the mother to "fail" to meet every need of her infant, allowing him to develop and progress. This must be done according to the baby and child's growing ability to manage such disruptions. A certain "failure" in attunement was necessary for the infant to establish a sense of separateness and for boundaries between self and other to form. Such "failures" or disruptions were also viewed as necessary to develop the capacity to tolerate frustration and uncertainty and to "go on being" despite it (Winnicott, 1963). In fact, Winnicott suggested that this capacity was essential in forming a solid sense of self.

In a similar vein, Winnicott (1963) suggested that the "good enough" therapist is one who also fails in ways that are tolerable to the patient, providing him the opportunity to grow in his ability to handle frustration, uncertainty, and imperfection – in other words – to self-regulate. "Self-regulation refers to an ability to engage in the world and experience a full range of emotions without falling apart." (Tronick & Gold, 2020, pp. 107–108). Of course, this requires the therapist to tolerate his own limitations, not always being liked and, in fact, welcoming the patient's anger and disappointment in response to frustration. This requires the creation of a holding environment in which all the patient's feelings are acceptable – even or perhaps especially, the messy and difficult ones.

The Necessity of Challenge and Disruption for Growth

Davanloo (1978, 1979, 1990) has long been an advocate for incorporating challenge into the therapeutic relationship. He abandoned the medical model, with its excessive focus on pathology, and developed a potential model in which therapist and patient are challenged to work at their highest level of capacity in order to heal, grow, and become their best selves. In contrast to the neutral stance often advocated by his psychoanalytic colleagues, he advocated taking a stand for growth and healing and against anything destructive. Once an alliance is established, with an agreement about problems, goals, and tasks, the patient is challenged to get to work immediately. This point must be reiterated. Challenge appears to be most effective within the context of a trusting relationship. Premature challenge or challenge in the absence of a solid therapeutic alliance often backfires.

Since excessive reliance on defenses against the patient's feelings, wishes, and desires most often causes, and certainly exacerbates their difficulties, we challenge the patient to abandon these avoidant strategies in favor of honesty with self and others. Challenging a patient's defenses often causes temporary disruption in the relationship – a disruption that is necessary for change. Davanloo (1990, 2000) is not alone in this approach. Reich (1949) advocated a challenge to the patient's defenses – or character armor, as he called it – which, left unattended, can become an impenetrable barrier to authentic connection and therapeutic change. Kohut (1984) suggested an atmosphere of "optimal frustration" in order to support "the patient's innate striving toward health and inborn ability to self-correct in the face of environmental perturbation" (p. 54).

More recently, Stark (1994, 2019) has been an advocate for the use of pressure to induce stress, which promotes growth and recovery from the suffering caused by resistance to change. In her words, "the therapist precipitates disruption in order to trigger repair...In this way we use pressure and induce stress to promote recovery" (p. 53). For this sort of intentional disruption to be experienced as reparative and healing, the therapist must: (1) "frustrate" the patient in an accurate and well-timed manner and (2) the patient must be able to absorb and respond to the therapist's challenge.

Clinical Examples

An example of this occurred in my practice just this week. In the third session, with an anxious and inhibited patient, her position as a helpless victim was challenged. Rather than join this 25-year-old woman in externalizing the cause of her suffering (an impossibly self-absorbed mother), an intrapsychic focus was maintained. The therapist suggested that the patient's anxiety and depression were not the direct result of anything her mother was or wasn't doing, but was actually an inside job. Specifically, I pointed out how the patient was ignoring her own feelings, needs, and desires by focusing exclusively on what she imagined was going on with her mother. Rather than face her feelings of rage and pain toward her mother, she dissolved into tears and maintained a helpless, victimized position. It was her difficulty in dealing with her own feelings *toward her mother* (and others, including the therapist) that was the real culprit. While the patient tacitly agreed with this assessment at the time, in the following session, she revealed that underneath her compliance was an adamant refusal to accept responsibility for her current plight. She went on to acknowledge feeling both angry with the therapist for refusing to sympathize with her as a victim and grateful that she had maintained a view of the patient as a competent adult, fully capable of dealing with her own feelings directly. This constituted a necessary disruption to the status quo and fortified the alliance, as well as catapulting her development forward.

As illustrated in the previous example, it is inevitable that patients will have strong mixed feelings toward the therapist who challenges their defenses. A part of the patient appreciates the vote of confidence expressed when he is challenged to operate from the best in him, but another part feels angry that his typical defenses are being called into question. Rather than avoid this, encouraging the patient to face, experience, and express all his feelings toward the therapist promotes therapeutic movement. If the therapist needs to be liked and viewed as only supportive, she will fail the patient and undermine the therapeutic process.

Transference, Projection, and the Possibility of Rupture

When patients transfer feelings and reactions from important figures from the past onto the person of the therapist, the alliance can suffer. Misalliance and rupture can result when the patient declares, "You are just like my mother," for example. Deft handling of these responses, in which distortions are corrected and feelings are faced, rather than avoided, is required to facilitate repair. Very often, there is a kernel of truth that must be acknowledged, while disentangling the distortions involved. In the following case, just such an interaction took place.

The Man Who Felt Guilty about Success

A 35-year-old single man came for help with anxiety and depression that had been triggered by the sale of his tech company for hundreds of millions of dollars. While consciously seeking success, and initially being thrilled by this bonanza, he quickly fell into a depression in which guilt over his success was a prominent feature. In an attempt to assuage that guilt, he gave a good deal of money to charity, and even built an orphanage in South America, all to no avail. He derived no satisfaction from these denotations and continued to be plagued by guilt about his riches.

Inquiry revealed that this was his second depressive episode. The first took place four years earlier when his girlfriend ended their relationship. He sought out therapy at that time but acknowledged being "skeptical and guarded" about the process. As a result, the treatment ended in failure.

A valued friend and colleague recommended the current therapist, so he decided to give it another try. Despite his conscious determination to get help, defenses against closeness were still in evidence and had to be addressed in order to prevent another useless treatment attempt.

TH: *It sounds like you are aware of two major difficulties – one is in understanding and dealing with your anxiety and guilt about winning and being successful, and the other is this conflict around closeness. You said that your girlfriend left you because she found you distant and only erratically available. You also acknowledged being distant, skeptical and guarded in your first attempt at therapy, which also failed.*

PT: *Yes, true. I am really baffled by this depressive reaction to my own success. I just feel guilty as hell, as if I don't deserve this. I want to understand that because I am miserable.*

TH: *So that is a clear goal – to get to the bottom of this – why you are so guilty about success and have to punish yourself with anxiety and depression. What about this other issue regarding closeness? How do you see that?*

PT: *Yes, in a way, it's a similar kind of ambivalence I get into. I want closeness and want the best girl, but when I get her, I back off. I feel I need my space and have this sense of being confined. I wanted my girlfriend badly, but then backed away and was devastated when she dumped me.*

TH: *Clearly there are intensely mixed feelings there and, again, some conflict about winning and letting yourself have and enjoy the spoils of victory.*

PT: *You go it.*

Patient and therapist were able to agree on the problems to be addressed and goals to be obtained in therapy. The patient was able to see a parallel between his difficulties in dealing with his business success and those in relationship to women. The next factor required to solidify the therapeutic alliance involved agreement about the therapeutic task.

While open and revealing in content, the patient appeared emotionally detached. He avoided the therapist's eyes and revealed no emotion, even while declaring that he was "devastated" by the loss of his previous girlfriend and "guilty" about his success. Furthermore, he acknowledged being distant and uninvolved in a previous therapy, which resulted in failure. To prevent yet another repetition of the need to fail, the transference pattern of behavior would have to be addressed and reversed. His response to this type of intervention was required to establish the therapeutic task.

TH: *Now, if we look at it, we see a similar pattern already in operation here with me. You want help and, in order to get help, you'll have to open up. You are physically present and cognitively involved but emotionally detached. You avoid my eyes and create a distance here. Do you see that?*

PT: *Well, I don't know you. It will take a while.*

TH: *And the question is how you are going to get to know me, and whether I can help you, if you keep yourself at arm's length. Is it just a matter of time or is this your pattern – to be half in and half out, to keep a certain distance and avoid intimacy and closeness?*

PT: *Well, I don't know. It seems pretty understandable to me that I would be anxious and wary – taking my time to get to know you.*

TH: *Again, the question is whether this is just what anyone would feel or whether this is an example of your pattern. How are you going to know if I can help you if you don't let me in? Will time alone resolve this? From what I understand, it only gets worse over time.*

PT: *That's true. With women, during the chase, I am all in and really go for it. It's only when she lets me know she's serious that I freak out.*

TH: *So we see you are keeping an emotional distance here with me and that doing so will result in failure, just like the last time. We know you are afraid to succeed for some reason and that you undermine your own goals and end up the loser.*

PT: *That's true.*

TH: *So is that what you want, or you are willing to open up to get help in resolving this?*

Before moving to the stage of pressure to feeling in the transference, the transference pattern of behavior, and it's parallel to identified problems in the patient's life, must be made clear. Then and only then is the patient in the position to make a choice to perpetuate an unhealthy pattern of relating or to do things differently. The patient's response to intervention will determine the next move. If he turns on the defenses against emotional engagement and opens up, we can follow the alliance. If he defends his defenses and increases his resistance, a head-on collision may be required.

PT: *This is so strange. Right before I sold the company, this guy tried to do a hostile takeover. He was really difficult to deal with and I was afraid I was losing control and he would just do a grab of what I had created. We had an intense conflict. I remember actually having the fantasy that he would kill me. I even saw myself getting beaten to death.*

This response is a clear message from the unconscious alliance, revealing deeper information about that nature of the conflict at hand. Given this, the therapist pursued more information on the current conflict, with the aim of helping him face his feelings toward his rival. It became clear that, for him, conflicts involve a battle to the death in which he must end up the loser. When he wins, he is filled with guilt, suggesting that triumph is associated, at least unconsciously, with him killing off and destroying his opponent. This is a hypothesis at this point and will have to be tested out over time.

TH: *Talk about being the loser! So he would kill you? What about your feelings toward him?*
PT: *He was an arrogant SOB!*
TH: *And your feelings toward him? He was trying to take over the company you build from scratch.*
PT: *It freaked me out.*
TH: *Let's see how you feel toward him.*
PT: *I feel anxious, almost like a panic.*
TH: *How do you experience that anxiety inside?*
PT: *It's that fight or flight thing. I am tense and feel hot and tingling, like energy surging through my body.*
TH: *Is that just anxiety or is there another feeling there? What is the feeling toward this guy?*
PT: *I guess I'm angry.*
TH: *You guess or you can feel anger, heat and energy surging through your body?*
PT: *Yeah, it's anger but also anxiety.*
TH: *That suggests you are terrified of your anger – like what might happen if you let yourself feel that toward him?*
PT: *I would want to kill him.*

TH: *How? What is the impulse, if this rage came out at him?*

PT: *I would smash his face in and kick him when he's down. He was so damn arrogant.*

TH: *So you can feel the impulse to smash his face, knock him down and kick him. What is the scene?*

PT: *There is blood everywhere, but now I want to kick him again.*

TH: *So there is more rage?*

PT: *It's like a sense of satisfaction. I see myself laughing.*

TH: *But I wonder what other feelings come then. On the one hand, it feels great and there is almost sadistic satisfaction in killing this guy, but how would you feel if you actually killed him. If you look into his face and his eyes, what do you see?*

PT: *His face is bashed in and it's very bloody.*

TH: *What color are his eyes?*

PT: *Blue-gray.*

TH: *Who has eyes like that?*

PT: *How strange – my Dad. I was close to my Dad growing up, but when I became a teenager, he changed. He was harsh with my Mom and me too. He started to tease me. We had this big, beautiful tree in our yard that I liked to climb. One day when I was about 13 he walked by and said, "Get out of that tree, you silly boy. That is childish". I felt full of shame. I think, at that moment, I decided to get tough.*

TH: *So, these conflicts about winning and losing – being a tough guy who dominates or a loser -may have started right there. What feelings do you have toward your father for shaming you?*

PT: *Angry. It's like with that other guy – he was arrogant and putting me down. I now see that I was furious and wanted to get them back. This all makes sense and I feel calm right now.*

It seemed as if the trial therapy went well. Acquainting the patient with his defenses against closeness in the transference, which would result in another failure if not removed, proved effective, at least temporarily. He opened up and revealed fresh material, shedding light on the origin of his conflict regarding competition, winning, and losing in relation to other men. However, when we began to explore his conflicts with women, the alliance was threatened with a possible rupture.

PT: *This really helps me begin to understand this guilt I have about winning and why I feel so guilty. I'm not nearly so clear about what is happening with women and why I sabotage my relationships.*

TH: *Is that what you would like to examine now?*

PT: *Yes. The fact is, I have more than enough money to live the rest of my life. I am sure I will want to work again but it doesn't seem so important right now. What I want more than anything is a great relationship with a woman and a family. I really want to get that sorted.*

TH: *How would you describe the problem?*

PT: *I get the woman I want and then I get bored. I can also start to feel hemmed in or intruded upon.*

TH: *Let's look at a recent example so we can clear on what is going on here.*

PT: *Like with my last girlfriend, as soon as I felt like I was falling in love – we went on this great trip together and made love. I felt close to her and then suddenly wanted to be on my own. When I realize this person could hurt me, I start to back off.*

TH: *Am I understanding this right – you get close, start to fall in love, and then worry you will lose the woman to someone else – she could leave you and hurt you?*

PT: *Yes.*

The question was whether he imaged he would be the loser to another man and would unconsciously need to arrange that (due to his guilt about winning), or had, in fact, been jilted in the past. In the latter case, if he had not dealt with his feelings about that rejection, he could project it into the future. Patients often worry that something *will* happen in the future that, in fact, has already happened. Working through feelings from the past so they are not repeated in the future is the task in that case. Inquiry was required to sort this out.

TH: *So, instead of projecting that into the future, did that already happen?*

PT: *That happened a lot in the early days. I got rejected a lot. My first girlfriend left me for another guy. I found her texting this other guy.*

TH: *Can we look at the feelings toward this girl? Can we have a first name?*

PT: *Pam. I really loved her. She was kind and sweet, smart and beautiful.*

TH: *But she was texting someone else when involved with you, is that right?*

PT: *Yeah, she was jerking me around.*

TH: *If you go back to the time when you discovered that, how do you feel toward Pam?*

PT: *I really loved her. She was my first love.*

TH: *And, from what you are saying, she betrayed you. How do you feel toward her?*

PT: *I felt awful. I was really crushed and so afraid she'd reject me.*

TH: *You were crushed and hurt by her, so what was the feeling toward her?*

PT: *It sounds like you want me to be angry with her, but I really loved her.*

It seemed as if we were headed for a possible rupture at this point in the process. The patient was angry with the therapist and, in the face of that anger, was projecting certain motives and characteristics onto her that, left unattended, would seriously undermine the therapeutic alliance. Pressing for feeling before clarification could backfire and further reinforce the notion that the therapist had her own agenda. Instead, the therapist decided to clarify the therapeutic task and bolster the alliance first.

TH: *Let's clear this up. You asked for my help in understanding these difficulties in relationship with women, right?*

PT: *Yeah.*

TH: *So, is it something I want or something you asked for?*

PT: *I asked for help, but I don't want you pushing me to be angry. I was really devastated and felt like a real loser when she dumped me for this other guy. Then I started to want to get tough and macho and guarded – like no one is going to hurt me.*

TH: *It sounds like you have a pretty good understanding of that part of it, and that makes sense. Still, you are having the same problems. What is missing are your reactive feelings toward Pam for hurting you.*

PT: *Now I am getting angry at you. I have this feeling you are taking over and trying to put your ideas on me. It's almost like you want your way and it's your way or the highway.*

The rupture seemed to be deepening. Rather than retreat or back pedal, the therapist persisted in trying to clarify what was taking place and to correct course by making sure the patient was the one deciding how to proceed.

TH: *Let's slow down and sort out what's happening here. As we start to examine your relationships and what is in the way, a history of being hurt and rejected by women has emerged. This is a topic you raised and asked to have my help with. So, I am responding to your request. At the same time, you see me as taking over and forcing my agenda. How do you understand this?*

PT: *Yes, I want to understand it and get it resolved, but I don't want you to railroad me.*

TH: *I did, in fact, bring up what appears to be a missing piece, which is your reactive feelings toward the women you love who hurt you. It is up to you – not me – to decide whether that is something you want to explore. You are aware of the hurt from the past and how you have tried to guard yourself against this by keeping an emotional distance. I think you are also beginning to see how that emotional distance is now contributing to the failure in your subsequent relationships with women. Your solution has become a problem it seems to me, but it's up to you to determine.*

As previously noted, in order to repair a rupture, it is necessary for the therapist to acknowledge her part and not simply lay the difficulty at the patient's feet. In so doing, we can also clarify the issue of causation. The therapist did, in fact, raise the issue of reactive feelings toward Pam. How the patient felt toward the therapist for raising this issue, and how he defended against those feelings, were separate matters that needed to be sorted out. Persistence seemed to pay off. By repeating that (1) the therapist said something, (2) the patient had a feeling and reaction to this, and (3) he was free to decide how to deal with that, not only cleared away the transference distortion but also led to a significant link to the past that helped us understand the distortion.

PT: *I just had this thought that you are trying to break my spirit.*
TH: *That's a very specific concern. What gives you that idea?*
PT: *I just realized this is how it felt with my mother. She was extremely judgmental and intrusive – always in my business and telling me what to do. I couldn't stand it.*
TH: *So there is a link between me and your mother.*
PT: *Well, I thought that was happening between us, but now I realize it's really about the relationship with my Mom. You were actually giving me a choice, with her, it was definitely her way or the highway. She would scream and holler and slap me into submission. You could not disagree with her.*

We were able to use a rupture-repair cycle to avert a misalliance and to further the process. Initially, a link was made between the therapist and the patient's mother. As soon as that became conscious, he was able to make a distinction between the two. We were then able to proceed to facing feelings toward his mother and other women, in an effort to help him resolve the conflicts he had been acting out. When resolved and repaired, alliance ruptures often lead to deeper and more lasting results, as was the case here.

Head-on Collision with the Resistance

The case of The Errant Priest proved to be quite complex, and therapeutic progress was erratic. Uncovering the original source of symptoms proved insufficient for their removal. In addition, identifying the various factors that sustained them was also required. In many ways, these behaviors had become functionally autonomous. In other words, they had become disconnected from their original source and took on a life of their own. Furthermore, developmental issues and characterological difficulties complicated the picture and added layers of complexity to the case.

When sent away to an isolated location with Priests who were all acting out sexually, he avoided his pain and rage via a process of identification – becoming like them. Of note, the patient could identify his emotions and the impulses associated with them, but tended to avoid the actual, visceral experience of these feelings. In this case, acting out was a compromise between the desire to express his anxiety-provoking and guilt-laden feelings while defending against the internal experience of them.

The early sessions seemed to be very effective in helping him understand the compulsive behavior that had completely perplexed him at the inception of treatment. Understanding their origins, and experiencing the feelings he had been avoiding, resulted in dramatic improvement. He was very pleased with his progress, and I was optimistic, expecting progress to continue apace. Then, bumps appeared in the road, and he started to relapse. A particular pattern of behavior emerged in which he would regress and act out after particularly helpful sessions (two steps forward and one step back). Since we had already delineated many of the negative consequences of his acting out, we began to explore whether there were some positive benefits to it as well. It became clear that he was starting to associate the resolution of his conflicts with the loss of the therapeutic relationship. Given this, a part of him was holding onto the relationship by being needy and troubled. In doing so, he could prolong therapy and avoid grief over loss. So, while this factor did not contribute to the initial development of the symptom, it became a factor in maintaining it.

Since the patient knew that he was avoiding feelings in ways that hurt him, but continued to behave in this destructive manner, a head-on collision with defenses that were now operating as a resistance to treatment was indicated. The patient was challenged to take a stand regarding his own destructiveness. In turn, the therapist acknowledged her own limits and refused to assume a dominant or omnipotent stance, underscoring the fact that therapeutic results could only be obtained with his will and engagement on board. Conversely, it was pointed out that the patient could destroy the therapist's efforts if he chose to do so. Making this clear and putting the ultimate choice in the patient's lap, while taking an unequivocal stand for health and healing and against anything destructive, is the essence of this powerful but difficult intervention.

PT: *I was so strong and happy the last time. Then, I do this thing. I am afraid I will destroy myself and there is nothing I can do about it.*

TH: *You have, in fact, destroyed that good feeling. You take a passive, helpless position in the face of your own destructiveness, as if you can't do anything about it. If you go passive, what will happen?*

PT: *It will just keep happening.*

TH: *In each instance you make a choice – to say yes or no – but in another way you sit on the fence – say one thing and do another. The fact is, you can't have it both ways. You are neither a single man nor a Priest.*

PT: *What should I do? I want to confront myself but maybe I am testing you. Will you throw me out?*

Patients often create interpersonal conflicts in order to avoid facing their internal conflicts. It seemed that the patient was trying to engage the therapist to take over, so he could stay in the passive, compliant/defiant position. Instead of responding to his demands, maintaining a focus on his internal conflict (in order to intensify it and create a crisis) was initiated. In the end, it must be made clear that the choice to face or avoid his true feelings was ultimately up to him.

TH: *What you do is your business. Asking me to take over is going to the passive position again. We are two people, and we have two choices. There is no reason to continue in this way – with you acting out and then confessing and asking for penance. I, for one, won't do it anymore. You are wanting to play it out, as if it is between us, when, in fact, it's between you and you. The only question is what you are going to do about this.*

This aspect of the head-on collision, in which the patient is held responsible for his own choices, while the therapist declares her own position, is crucial. Therapists often engage with, and continue to treat, anyone willing to come to their office and pay their fee, regardless of how the patient is making use of the therapy. Doing so can create a collusive alliance. In contrast, taking a stand for health and healing, and against anything destructive, is essential in solidifying a therapeutic alliance and challenging resistance that will undermine it.

PT: *I want to be free and to have real contact with real people. I don't really want others to decide for me. It's up to me to stop. Otherwise, it's a waste of time.*
TH: *What are your options? Where is the line for you?*
PT: *I have decided certain things, like sex without a condom is not an option and drugs are not an option, so on some level, having sex – servicing men – is still an option.*

The patient honestly acknowledged that he hadn't drawn a line in the sand for himself when it came to seeking out men for sexual liaisons. As long as that was the case, and the defense of acting out was an option, it had become, in essence, a resistance in the treatment. Until and unless the patient was committed to the process of real change in his life, no substantial progress would be made, and another therapy would result in failure. This is the essential truth that the head-on collision is designed to communicate.

TH: *As long as it's an option, it will continue, and as long as that is the case, we will get nowhere. We have focused a great deal on the destructive part of you, and the part of you that is hurt and gets victimized, but we now see there is a third element -- the silent co-conspirator – the part of you that knows what's going on and stands by passively, doing nothing about it.*

PT: *Like what happened with my mother. No one said no – don't go in his room – he has to grow up.*

TH: *No one did then, and now you don't. When will you take on that authority? You have a decision to make. You know what this is about, but you keep doing it anyway. There is no reason to continue, as if we are both dedicated to your freedom, when a part of you is still devoted to imprisonment.*

PT: *You're right. I really have to decide.*

TH: *Call me when you have made a firm decision. Continuing in this way is contributing to the problem.*

In addition to emotional conflicts regarding sexuality and anger, and the patient's characteristic pattern of passivity, compliance, and subservience, developmental issues emerged as significant factors in this case and needed to be addressed. This man was a good, submissive boy to his single mother, behaving more like a partner and husband than a son. He repressed his own feelings, needs, and desires and was compliant with hers. At 17, he fled his home to join the Seminary. In many ways, his personal development stopped at that point and was arrested in a sort of perpetual childhood. He had stayed a "mama's boy" and never went through a period of adolescent rebellion, often necessary to separate and individuate.

While having experienced a call from God at an early age, he also felt that becoming a Priest was the only acceptable way to separate from his mother. He essentially went from his mother's home to a "father's home," the Church. Again, he took a submissive and compliant position as a seminarian, being "good" and fitting into an existing structure and order.

It seemed increasingly apparent that, when his dear friend and mentor died (a man who exemplified all that was good about the Church), he flipped from compliance to defiance, and acted out in a way that represented a delayed period of adolescent rebellion. He had simply shifted from a pattern of sacrificing self to fit in with and please others, to doing whatever he wanted, with little regard for the needs and feelings of others. He was either doing to, or being done by the other, but there was no mutuality or reciprocity involved in these relationships. This is typical in cases of the repetition compulsion – in which one invites punishment (is the victim) or punishes others (perpetrator). In this case, he alternated between the two patterns of interaction.

Beyond mere symptom removal, the therapeutic task in this case included helping the patient to discover and solidify an authentic sense of self so that he could relate to others in a genuine fashion. The therapeutic relationship became a vehicle for his development, in which the compliant/defiant mode of relating was replaced with collaboration between two separate, but connected, human beings. Rather than schedule another session while he was in an ambivalent state, I told him to call me when he was ready. This "head-on collision" with the resistance proved effective. He contacted me a week later and said he was ready to go all-in and was determined to stop behaving in a destructive fashion.

Next Session

PT: *I was in shock after the last session. A part of me was angry with you for confronting me, but then it dawned on me that you are taking me, and this situation, very seriously. In a way, you were like a good father – not the permissive mother – but a father who can say no and urge me to "stand up" and "get going". No one ever said "no" to me, and I wasn't saying "no" to myself. Suddenly it seemed like a clear decision. I also see I have continued to act out to keep the therapy going – abandoning myself to hold onto you. Something changed internally. I know what I want to do. I almost felt ecstatic. Ever since that day, I have felt strong and have been praying, reading, putting my energy into healthy activities, and feeling happy and peaceful.*

TH: *This has happened before, so what is different? What has changed in you?* (This patient was a good talker and could say all the right things while failing to change his actual behavior. The therapist challenged him to act in accordance with his intentions).

PT: *I have never felt this way in my life. I have made a decision – to stop acting out. I really hadn't done that before. There was huge peace and relief in it. The decision was not just – or even mostly – about not acting out. It was a decision to stay a Priest. It was almost overwhelming. It's a very special and privileged position (*positive approach goal, as opposed to an avoidant one).

TH: *I wonder if you almost had to create a crisis to get to this point.*

PT: *Yes! I was destroying myself. It feels so different now.*

TH: *How did this happened?*

PT: *It's about my integrity. I think I've internalized you in a positive way. I see your face when I'm alone. You are always with me. Instead of defying you, it is a source of power and integrity. I have been mediating and praying a lot and have no doubts about my vocation.*

Research has confirmed that being in an acute crisis increases motivation and bodes well for a rapid response to treatment. In this case, the patient had been in a state of chronic despair for years. Therefore, the therapist needed to intervene in such a way as to create an internal crisis, by challenging him to stand up to his own destructiveness and do something different. When, despite his awareness of the destructive patterns that created and perpetuated his misery, he continued to rely on defense and avoidance, the therapist created an intentional disruption in the relationship by employing a head-on collision with the resistance in the transference. His response to this intervention suggested that just such a disruption was both necessary and therapeutic.

Summary

In this chapter, we have reviewed the literature on rupture and repair in therapeutic relationships. Perhaps surprisingly, research suggests that relationships in which there are cycles of rupture and repair are stronger and more resilient than those that seem to run smoothly, but are never tested. That said, ruptures to the alliance that are ignored and not repaired contribute to the failure of therapeutic efforts. Clinical examples of both intentional ruptures and those created unintentionally were included.

Chapter 7

Autonomy and Attachment

In "Civilization and its Discontents" (1930/1961), Freud wrote that "the development of the individual seems...to be a product of the interaction between two urges" – to attach and to individuate (p. 140). He noted that these two drives were often in conflict, warring for supremacy. Correspondingly, Freud outlined two major sources of anxiety – the fear of loss of love and the fear of punishment, regarding guilt over aggressive urges. Throughout life, we all confront two developmental challenges: "a) to establish and maintain reciprocal, meaningful, and personally satisfying interpersonal relationships and b) to establish and maintain a coherent, realistic, differentiated, integrated, essential positive sense of self" (Blatt, 2008, p. 3). Psychological development is largely concerned with establishing balance and integration of these two basic human needs. Over time, we may shift from an emphasis on one to the other yet, in health, attending to both needs, such that the more solid the sense of self, the better one is able to attach. Conversely, the more securely attached, the freer one is to explore separateness.

In this way, "psychopathology can be understood as distorted, exaggerated, one-sided preoccupations....with normal developmental issues of interpersonal relatedness or self-definition" (Blatt, 2008, p. 5).

Most often, we see patients who sacrifice self in a desperate attempt to secure attachments to others. These patients are anxious and preoccupied with the state of their relationships and tend to be passive, dependent, subservient, and compliant with the needs and wishes of others in order to maintain the relationship. These individuals are especially vulnerable to depression when relationships falter or end. The fear of being unloved, unwanted, and uncared for is primary. They are most likely to develop what Blatt (2008) has referred to as anaclitic depression.

More rarely, therapists see those who give up on relationships in order to hold onto themselves. These patients are more likely to be obsessional, schizoid, paranoid, or narcissistic. They are preoccupied with maintaining a positive sense of self at all costs, discarding relationships that don't feed their need for mirroring. They are most concerned with feelings of inadequacy, guilt, and failure. This group suffers from what Blatt (2008) calls

DOI: 10.4324/9781003197669-7

introjective depression; often following a failure to achieve desired goals and aspirations.

Not only do these two "types" of individuals develop different sorts of depression, but Blatt's research findings have suggested that these two groups experience the therapeutic encounter very differently as well (Blatt, Besser & Ford, 2007; Blatt & Shahar, 2004; Blatt & Zuroff, 2005). The anaclitic group tends to respond best to supportive interventions, while the introjective group typically responds most therapeutically to experiential and interpretive interventions.

Of interest, results from the Mental Health-Sponsored Treatment of Depression Collaborative Research Program (Elkin et al., 1985) found that the self-criticism characteristic of the introjective patient often impedes the therapeutic process, suggesting that long-term therapy is the best option. However, rapid and sustained focus on the defense of self-attack can ameliorate its destructive impact on treatment efforts and speed the process of healing (Abbass, 2015; Coughlin Della Selva, 2004; Frederickson, 2013).

Over the past several decades, our field has been preoccupied with the issue of attachment. As a result, we may have neglected to focus on the importance of helping patients develop a solid but flexible and autonomous sense of self as well, the other pillar of well-being.

Consolidating an Integrated Sense of Self

> Human beings are not born once and for all on the day their mothers give birth to them, but that life obliges them over and over to give birth to themselves.
>
> Gabriel Garcia Marquez

As James Mann (1991) has reminded us, our patients are often stuck in existential time, with the sense that their "chronically and presently endured pain" will remain forever fixed. It's as if their damaged view of self is frozen in time – has always has been, is now, and always will be going forward. This negative view of self inevitably involves the sense of being a victim. "The childhood victimization tends to become perpetuated as a guiding fiction in the life of an adult" (Mann, 1991, p. 20). Since this constitutes a deeply held belief, it can become self-perpetuating and self-fulfilling. The following case is a prime example of this kind of dynamic.

The Worrier

A 60-year-old woman came for help with anxiety, panic, various pain syndromes, and a tendency to worry incessantly about negative events that might occur sometime in the future. She viewed herself as helpless in the face of life's vicissitudes and reported an overtly critical inner dialog, which inevitably led to depressive affect. These symptoms were nearly lifelong. She had despaired of getting better, as many rounds of previous psychotherapy had proved ineffective. Somehow, she came upon Howard Schubiner's (Schubiner & Beltzolt, 2010) work, looked on his website, and decided to engage an Intensive Short-Term Dynamic Psychotherapy (ISTDP) practitioner, a treatment with empirical evidence as effective with somatic symptoms and treatment-resistant depression (Abbass, 2015).

Inquiry revealed that she was the youngest in a large brood, and the only girl in her family. To fit in, she tried to be something she was not – a rough and tumble boy. This tendency to deny herself and mold herself into a shape that might secure an attachment to others had a devastating effect on her life. In fact, she had gone so far as to have affairs with both a priest and a therapist; so desperate was she to give them whatever they wanted in exchange for some semblance of care. Her sense of herself as worthless was profound. To resolve her difficulties, it proved necessary but insufficient to help her access rage toward those who used and abused her. We needed to unveil her unconscious beliefs about herself so they could be altered. This could be summed up as, "I must prostitute myself in order to get others to pay attention to me. I must give up my own needs and feelings to meet those of others, lest I be abandoned. I am utterly forgettable."

In a pivotal session, she allowed herself to experience anger toward someone in her current life who had not responded to her bid for connection. Underneath the anger was searing pain. Suddenly she saw herself as an infant in a crib, utterly alone. When she was ten months old, her mother fell ill and had to be hospitalized for several weeks. Her father had to work and couldn't care for all the children in the family, so she was taken to an orphanage until her mother recovered. Of course, three to four weeks is an eternity to an infant. Without any way to understand what was transpiring, she was taken from her home and everyone she knew and loved, while left alone in a strange and sterile place. Clearly, the sense that she was forgettable, and that loved ones could simply disappear, leaving her alone and destitute, was deeply embedded in her psyche.

PT: *Oh my God. That's it – that's what happens every time someone I need and love doesn't respond. It's like I'm a desperate infant again. I'm back there in that crib – alone, desperate, and utterly helpless.*

TH: *But you're not.*

The session was over, so no more could be said. Yet, she began the next session by revealing how important that deceptively simple statement was for her.

PT: *Three words! "But you're not." "But you're not." I can't tell you how many times that awareness came to me during the past week. I am no longer a helpless infant. I am a capable adult. It has been life changing.*

I was completely taken by surprise, as my comment did not strike me as particularly profound at the time. However, for her, it somehow helped her shift into the present time. She had been living in a kind of time warp – thinking and feeling as if she was completely helpless, like an infant, with no sense of agency in getting her needs met in relationships. Her whole sense of self was dramatically altered by this experience. It was the sort of juxtaposition that Ecker (Ecker et al., 2012) suggests is pivotal in the process of change. While it may be tempting to think there was something magical about those three words, it was one of many factors involved in her healing. That said, it was a powerful experience that had a lasting impact on her sense of self.

It bears repeating that, in order to effect change in the patient's sense of self, helping her experience previously avoided feelings toward others proved necessary, but insufficient for change. As long as she viewed herself as a desperate and dependent infant (even as a 60-year-old woman), she would do anything to please or appease those who were important to her. "The way a person assesses ongoing lived time is determined by how he or she perceives personal adequacy in the face of some challenging reality" (Mann, 1991, p. 17). In many cases, including the one cited here, this sense of self-efficacy (or lack thereof) is based on the past – an outmoded sense of self that leads to anxiety and depression. Our interventions are designed to help the patient face the past in order to achieve some mastery over it in the present time and, in so doing, free her to shape a new future.

A Woman Unfulfilled

A 63-year-old woman contacted me shortly after the death of her parents and the birth of her first grandchild. The pull to become a caretaker to the new baby (as she had done in her family of origin), rather than finally pursuing her own dreams, prompted a crisis and motivated her to finally reach out for help.

TH: *How can I help?*
PT: *I have never gone for therapy before but feel it's time.*
TH: *What are your concerns?*
PT: *I'm 63. My parents recently died (starts crying). What is wrong with me?*
TH: *Some feelings are coming up as you mention their deaths.*
PT: *I miss them.*
TH: *But you also criticize yourself for having these feelings. Are you aware that you are anxious?*
PT: *Yes – very. It's the idea of being vulnerable. As the oldest of 5, I was always pretending to be the strong one. I am not used to being vulnerable or asking for help.*
TH: *How do you experience this anxiety about opening up and being vulnerable?*
PT: *Overheating. I feel a lot of tension in my solar plexus.*

TH: *You get anxious about these painful feelings, tense up, and then feel constricted in your chest.*

PT: *Yes (big smile).*

TH: *And you smile. Is this another way to avoid being vulnerable by covering up and pretending everything is OK?*

To maximize effectiveness, both the assessment of anxiety, and the identification of defenses used to avoid the feelings that trigger anxiety, begins as soon as these patterns are in evidence. The patient's response to these early interventions largely determines the pace and course of subsequent treatment efforts. In this case, the patient proved highly responsive.

PT: *Definitely. There was that in my family. You might be Irish too – and know something about this – put on a happy face, don't complain, you're blessed and all that. And, of course, I am. I am almost embarrassed to be asking for help. So many have it worse. You know that attitude is OK sometimes, but there are times I need to look at what's underneath it all.*

The patient was already catching her own defenses of minimization and rationalization and turning on them – a good sign. She was aware of anxiety about the process of opening up, being vulnerable, and daring to ask for help. Since she had spent her life complying with family dictates to be strong, to smile, and always make the best of things, defying these dictates was experienced as quite threatening. At the same time, she was determined to stop this pattern. The activation of the conflict between the patient's deepest feelings and desires and the unconscious prohibitions against them precipitated a crisis and prepared the way for deep and rapid change.

TH: *And that's why you're here.*

PT: *Yes.*

TH: *Are you actually from down South?*

PT: *This is where the story begins. I was born in New York to Irish immigrants. Weirdly, my grandparents took me back to Virginia from the ages of 2 to 4. Then we all moved back in with my parents until I was 6. I remember it like it was yesterday. They all took me out to dinner, which was very rare, and asked me if I wanted to go back to the farm with Granddad. I said I would love to because I was incredibly close to him from the start. Even as a little girl, I caught a glimpse of pain in my father's face when I said yes (starts to cry). So I moved down south and stayed there until the age of 14.*

TH: *With your grandfather?*

PT: *Both my grandparents. I had an idyllic childhood on their farm, but I was separated from my family. I wasn't suffering. I was loved and protected.*

TH: *How do you understand it?*

PT: *My mother was an only child. My grandmother had a boy afterward, but he died at the age of 4. Then she had a string of still births. My mother had 5 children in 6 years. I think my mother wanted to give her mother a child. She sacrificed me to fill a void in her mother's life, who had always wanted a big family, but couldn't have one. They were delighted to have me, but I was left wondering, "Who am I – am I my mother's baby sister or her first child?"*

TH: *This had to be incredibly confusing as well as deeply upsetting.*

PT: *I went back to New York for the summer when I was 10, 12, and 14. At the end of that last summer, my mother asked me if I wanted to stay with them or go back to the farm. I was thriving in Virginia but living in New York City was so exciting. I was a teenager, so cars and boys and going out for burgers was very appealing. My parents were musicians and very well-known at this point. Our home was a magnet – it was the place to be – where everyone gathered. At the same time, I knew I shouldn't stay.*

TH: *What do you mean?*

PT: *I let my grandfather down and he died shortly thereafter.*

TH: *What happened?*

PT: *He died of a heart attack. It's all very complex. My grandmother was very ambitious and quite successful. She was elegant, regal, and rather showy – appearances meant a lot. My mother ended up getting pregnant with me out of wedlock and she thought her mother would be furious. They got married quickly and ran off, not telling anyone about the baby. Then, her father was hospitalized, and it looked like he was going to die. She had to decide to keep the secret and stay away or take the baby – me – and go to the hospital, so that's what she did. When she arrived at the hospital, her mother was so thrilled with the baby she couldn't care less about the time-line. The story goes that Granddad was dying of heart disease. They put me on his chest, and he miraculously recovered. There were even stories about it in the newspaper.*

TH: *So, there was this dramatic story and a powerful connection between you and your granddad from the start.*

PT: *Right, as if I had saved him. Then when I said I would stay with my parents, it killed him. Intellectually, I know this isn't true, but if I had only stayed with him (crying)! Why were boys and cheeseburgers so important? I didn't even have my own room in New York and had to sleep on the couch. I blamed myself and no longer trusted myself to make decisions. I hurt my dad when I went to Virginia and hurt my grandfather when I stayed in New York. Intellectually I know I shouldn't have been asked to make these decisions.*

It was becoming clear that the patient avoided her own feelings and complied with the wishes of others. In addition, she blamed herself for any and all negative outcomes that befell herself or others. This suggested a pattern of repressing her own anger and turning it back on herself. That hypothesis was tested out in the following sequence.

TH: *You understand that intellectually but what about your feelings about being put in these impossible situations repeatedly?*

PT: *It was awful. I also disrupted the family when I came back home. My younger brother had been king of the castle. He resented me. Then I remember my sister saying, "Are you my sister? I thought you were my cousin."*

TH: *Your parents gave you up and over to your grandparents and didn't even keep you alive in their memory. You must have all kinds of feelings toward them.*

PT: *Here's the thing. I'm busy not making anyone wrong.*

TH: *Except you. You blame yourself, as if your decisions were the problem. What about your feelings toward them for putting you in these situations?*

PT: *I love my mother, father, grandmother, and grandfather. They loved me, but it doesn't mean it was right.*

We were able to observe the ways in which the patient had abandoned herself, as she was abandoned, and continued to sacrifice her own needs, feelings, and wishes in order to care for others. She was fiercely protective of her family and was willing to take it on the chin rather than face her angry feelings toward them. However, the death of her parents and birth of a grandchild precipitated a crisis in which she was ready to face what she had been avoiding all her life. She did not want to die never having lived, with her unique gifts and contribution still under wraps. Her goal was to become more self-directed and self-validated, rather than relying excessively on an other-validated sense of self.

At first, she declared that she felt lost and had no idea what she needed or wanted to do with her life. For some reason, this didn't ring true. The therapist had the sense that the patient knew what she wanted but was afraid to declare it. Again, this hunch was tested out and confirmed.

TH: *You say you are lost and have no idea what you want to do with your life, but I sense that isn't true.*

PT: *You're right. I am a writer and have already started a documentary, a novel, and even have a clear idea for a television series. I would love to do this more than anything (starts to cry). I want to be valued for who I am.*

TH: *Which means you would have to reveal it – to be real rather than just complying with the demands of others.*

PT: *That's it exactly and that's why I've come to you.*

TH: *Now it is clear you know exactly what you want to do but you are blocked. There are obstacles in the way.*

PT: *It's as if I have no right. A memory is coming to me. I have never relayed this to anyone. When I came home for the summer at the age of 12 my mother picked me up in this big car. She sat me beside her, in between her and my brother. Already I was taking up his spot. I could feel his resentment, though I had never experienced anything like it.*

TH: *You had been the one and only in Virginia.*

PT: *Also, there was never any sarcasm or unspoken subtext in our conversations. We had no TV or phone over there, so I was really naïve. He was very sarcastic and started goading me, asking me about my ability to sing and perform. They were all acting and singing from an early age – something I had never done. I felt hurt (starting to cry). Then, there's another memory. Geez, this is weird. This is probably where it all started. I was 14 and still sleeping on the sofa. A reporter came to the house to do a story about the children. We all sat down, but then they said to me, "No, we only want the siblings." I was asked to leave the room. They only wanted to talk to the people that mattered. I was the Princess on the farm, but there I was dethroned.*

The patient's conscious and unconscious alliance were very strong, brining material to be examined which helped us understand the origin of her conflicts, including those regarding rivalry and competition with her siblings.

TH: *These memories followed my asking about what is blocking you from realizing your own dreams and ambitions, and the theme of competition arises. Not everyone will applaud you if you get in the front seat. They might want to push you out. You have avoided this competition and all your feelings about it like the plague.*

PT: *God, you're good. That's so true. My brother is a good guy. How can I say this nicely?*

TH: *Why nicely? Can we have an honest look at your thoughts and feelings toward him?*

PT: *He's like Trump.*

TH: *A narcissist you mean?*

PT: *Thanks for saying it for me.*

TH: *But ultimately that won't help. Let's see what you say, and how you truly feel toward him.*

PT: *That's so strange. I can stand up to any other person or group. I don't take shit from people, and I can be fierce. However, in my family, I let them get away with murder. This need to fit in is the culprit.*

TH: *And how do you feel toward him?*

PT: *I am very angry, but I don't want to spend my time ruminating about that. I want to get rid of it.*

TH: *Isn't that the problem – all you do to avoid these feelings – and the price you pay for that. How can you own your own power and channel it into creativity when you are so anxious and guilty about it? The avoidance of your anger regarding competition keeps you in this hidden, one down position.*

PT: *You're right. Now I see it clearly.*

TH: *Is that what you want? To protect everyone else and sacrifice yourself in order to avoid these painful truths and your honest feelings about them, or to be real, authentic and self-expressed?*

PT: *I do. I am tired of being a ping pong ball, being tossed from one place to the next. Now, this is why I am here. I am not going to repeat this and just become the devoted grandmother. I want to do what I want to do. Of course, I am close to my children and want that with my grandchild, but not to give up my life to do so. I actually feel motivated to start writing, which is exciting.*

This patient was highly motivated to make changes and did so quickly. There was essentially no resistance to my interventions. She took everything I offered and ran with it. In fact, as the result of our work together, all the energy that had been bound up in the suppression of her feelings and desires was freed up and channeled into creativity. Not only was she able to face the feelings she had been avoiding, particularly toward her mother and brother, but was able to relinquish the back seat and take her place in the world by speaking (and writing!) in her own true voice. At the culmination of therapy, she was in the midst of filming a documentary and was well on her way to completing a memoir, which seemed to pour out of her once her need to suppress her feelings and the painful memories associated with them was no longer in operation.

This woman had spent 63 years renouncing her true self in order to attach to others, who demanded compliance and subservience. Her self-negation was both a manifestation of identification with depriving attachment figures and served as punishment for rage over the way she was being treated. Given the nature of the trauma to her early attachments, and the stories of how she both saved others by her presence and killed them when asserting her own desires, the tenacity of this pattern was understandable. The death of her parents, shortly followed by the birth of her first grandchild, precipitating an internal crisis between her desire to finally focus on her own wishes and desires and the internal pressure to suppress those in order to resume a caretaking role.

We are most likely to see patients who choose a relationship with others over their own interests and concerns. They are prone to anxiety, depression, and self-criticism. The pattern of people pleasing, compliance, and subservience, along with internal demands to be better, nicer, and kinder when things don't go well, are legend in this group. In contrast, those who sacrifice relationships in an effort to bolster their flagging self-esteem, prioritizing their own needs and wishes over those of others, are typically narcissistic and even sociopathic in their character and rarely seek our help voluntarily.

Schizoid and avoidant patients, who relinquish relationships due to excessive anxiety about close contact with others, are more likely to seek our help. In either case, the consequences of choosing one of these primary needs for the other is a prescription for misery.

Sacrificing Connection in Bid for Autonomy

Patients who sacrifice the need for connection in order to maintain their shaky sense of self are far more difficult to treat, particularly in a short period of time. In my experience, there are two types of patients who sacrifice relationships to maintain autonomy. The first group is highly anxious and avoidant. They long for the closeness of a primary relationship but become highly anxious, overwhelmed, and dysregulated when in close contact with others. As a result, they tend to give up on having the love they crave.

The other group tends to be cold and dismissive regarding needs for closeness. They prize their independence and tend to be narcissistic and, at times, even sociopathic. Unlike the anxious type who longs for closeness, while also fearing the intense feelings closeness engenders, the dismissive type denies any such longings. They use people for what they can get out of the transaction and avoid genuine emotional involvement. These patients tend to be quite self-satisfied and are often referred by others, who find them difficult to deal with. We'll begin with the anxious – avoidant type.

The Man Who Considered Himself a Basket Case

This 50-year-old single professional male came for help in order to understand and overcome intense conflicts regarding closeness, particularly with women. While longing for closeness and wanting to get married and have children, he was highly anxious around women and found himself incapable of initiating contact with them. As a result, the few short relationships he had had were all initiated by the woman. As soon as he got romantically involved, he would become completely preoccupied with the woman and flooded with anxiety and emotions he wasn't able to regulate. Consequently, he thought of himself as "a basket case." Furthermore, he would precipitously end the relationship in order to return to some state of stability. Shame would ensue and create further motivation to avoid trying (and, he assumed, failing) with women once again. In fact, it had been many years since he had had a relationship of any sort. While the restrictions of Covid eased the internal pressure to socialize, as they began to lift, his desire to resolve this conflict so that he could establish a lasting relationship had motivated him to seek treatment.

As with many highly avoidant patients, this man's conflict regarding closeness becomes clear in the transference relationship, where it was addressed directly. In this sense, patients show us what they may not be able to tell us directly. Having established agreement about the problems to be addressed and goals for therapy, we embarked upon the process of examining the transference pattern of behavior.

TH: *How are you feeling as we begin today?*
PT: *Tense in my shoulders (looks away).*
TH: *So there is anxiety and tension. You also look away and create some distance here, are you aware of that?*
PT: *Now that you mention it, yes.*
TH: *This is the very pattern that causes you problems in your life – you want connection but avoid it.*
PT: *I don't mean to but it's very automatic. I try to look at you but it's very uncomfortable.*
TH: *What happens when you make a connection here and actually look at me?*
PT: *I get spacey.*
TH: *Your anxiety is so high that it all starts to feel a bit unreal?*
PT: *Yes, it's like it used to be when I tried to speak to a woman – I would just space out and couldn't think of a word to say.*
TH: *As if you are terrified of closeness with a woman* (the patient had reported a number of close male friendships, so this conflict seemed to be restricted to women).
PT: *(sigh) I'm not sure why.*
TH: *You just sighed. Is the anxiety coming down? How is your thinking?*
PT: *Yes, it's a bit clearer now, but my stomach is tight, and I feel tension in my jaw.*

Initially, the patient's anxiety was so high he couldn't think straight. However, as we focused on the experience of his anxiety, it started to decrease in intensity. Sighing respiration and muscle tension, both cardinal signs of striated anxiety, were in evidence. This suggested that feelings were rising and that he might be able to tolerate them without going over his anxiety threshold.

TH: *Clamping down on your jaw? I wonder what feeling is coming up there toward me that you are keeping inside?*
PT: *(laughs) Well, you know, there is something about being with a powerful woman – I am not in control.*
TH: *So you see me as a powerful woman and are having a feeling toward me?*
PT: *There's an impulse to push back.*
TH: *And what's the feeling associated with that impulse?*
PT: *Anger.*
TH: *Can you feel that in your body?*
PT: *Yes, it's like an energy and I can feel heat rising.*
TH: *In your imagination, if that anger came out toward me, what do you see happening?*

PT: *Pushing you on your shoulders. I would smash you against the door.*
TH: *What would happen to me?*
PT: *You'd crumple on the floor.*
TH: *If you look at my face, what do you see?*
PT: *Vulnerability. Hurt. Dazed. Quiet. Now I feel guilty. This is what frightens me. I get so upset, what if I lash out and destroy the thing?*
TH: *Has that ever happened?*
PT: *No. I have never laid a hand on anyone. When that last relationship ended, I got terribly depressed.*
TH: *Might that be a way that you punish yourself due to your own guilt?*
PT: *I am just afraid it will all come out in an unregulated manner.*
TH: *And yet it doesn't. You protect the other from your anger and it goes back in on you. In a way, you have been living in solitary confinement ever since that relationship ended.*
PT: *This is very strange. I feel a kind of relief, having experienced all this. Now I can really see that I was furious with her. If I go back to that moment when she cut me off, I could rip her head off.*

As he experienced his true feelings and impulses, the unconscious opened, anxiety disappeared, and crucial information from the unconscious surfaced.

TH: *You can see this and feel it in your body?*
PT: *Yes. It's so strange. Now I am thinking of my mother. I suppose she was the original powerful woman in my life. She was very controlling and demanding. If I ever had a feeling or reaction, she would be appalled, "How dare you speak to me this way?" and crumple into tears.* (Notice the same word – crumpled – to refer to me and his mother.) *On the one hand she seemed very strong and commanding, but on the other hand she could dissolve into tears over the smallest push back.* (Again, the word "push" in regard to his impulse toward me and his mother.)
TH: *Clearly, you've been carrying around a lot of rage toward her, as well as guilt about this rage. The ultimate punishment has been to deprive yourself of what you most want – a warm, loving relationship with a woman. We can also see that getting close here with me, or with any woman, seems to stir up these feelings that create such anxiety and guilt.*
PT: *It is starting to make a kind of sense to me now.*

While this was just the start of the work that would take months to complete, working in the transference was crucial to success, and provided a direct route to the source of his conflicts around closeness with women. Just talking about external situations from a detached position would be of no therapeutic value. If the patient is using the same distancing defenses with the therapist that he employs in life, the same results will transpire, and failure will ensue. In this case, the patient's conflict was apparent in the transference relationship, where it was taken up directly. His willingness to abandon defenses and open up emotionally had a marked impact, both on the therapeutic relationship and his relationship with others. In fact, following this session, he reported having spoken openly and honestly about his feelings to his older sister, something he never would have done previously.

Cold, Detached, and Dismissive Patients

Unlike the anxious and avoidant patient just described, patients who deny any need or desire for closeness with others, while focusing on their own needs, feelings, and ambitions often come across as cold, arrogant, and narcissistic. They tend to be emotionally distant and highly dismissive of others and their attempts to establish a close bond. They jump in and out of relationships without much concern for the needs and feelings of the other. The fantasy that they can simply pop into therapy for a short course and leave without having to attach is more often a manifestation of their pathology than a healthy striving for healing. Research suggests that the development of an attachment to the therapist is a long and difficult process and, in large part, constitutes the bulk of the work in these cases (Kernberg, 1995; Yeomans & Caligor, 2016).

In reviewing my own work, four such cases stand out as rather colossal failures. These were all very attractive and highly successful men in their 40s. They had made millions and were adored by many from a distance. While they had many women at their beck and call, none had developed close or lasting relationships with anyone. In each case, someone else had suggested they get therapy. It is typically those in relationship with narcissists who suffer. These referrals are made in the vain hope that some changes might take place.

These men are often revered for their success. All too often, others let them get away with outrageous and demeaning behavior due to their "genius." Steve Jobs was a striking example of this phenomenon (Isaacson, 2011). He was abusive to employees, screaming and swearing at them for the slightest misstep. Apparently, these outbursts were tolerated for quite some time due to his extraordinary talents. However, even in his case, the consequences for such behavior eventually caught up to him, and he was fired by the very company he had founded. In my experience, it is only once the patient suffers such blows in the real world, that any possibility of change exists.

Typically, these men (there are obviously women with the same kind of character structure but, for whatever reason, I have not seen them in my practice) exhibit little motivation to look at themselves in an honest way and often externalize the source of the problems they encounter. Establishing an alliance and achieving agreement about problems, goals, and tasks is rarely accomplished in the short term with these patients. Instead, regular sessions over a more extended period of time (1–2 years) are typically required to achieve genuine character change in these cases (such as "The Cold-Blooded Businessman" in Coughlin Della Selva, 2004).

The Successful Loner

This 46-year-old single professional man traveled a significant distance in order to participate in a block therapy (two 2-hour sessions during each of two successive days). Since little information was obtained ahead of time, the therapist was not aware of how little internal motivation was present.

TH: *So tell me what brings you and how I can help.*
PT: *Well I'm not sure really. When I sold my company, they got a new CEO to take over and the feedback to me was that I am difficult and need to get some coaching or something.*
TH: *So you are responding to feedback and suggestions from others? If that hadn't happened, do you think you would be seeking help?*
PT: *Probably not – at least not at this time – and probably not for work issues. From my point of view, I have been very successful.*
TH: *Clearly you are successful on some level. You developed a business that was purchased?*
PT: *Yeah, it was super successful and sold for hundreds of millions.*
TH: *Yet they are letting you know there is some kind of problem – with your performance or what?*
PT: *Not my performance but the way I interact with others.*
TH: *What, in particular?*
PT: *I have no patience for people, and I guess I can get arrogant and testy.*
TH: *Is that a concern for you?*
PT: *Not really. I don't need employees to like me. I am not there to be their friend.*

Since the patient was clearly not concerned about his behavior in the workplace, other areas of functioning were explored in an attempt to agree on a therapeutic focus for the work.

TH: *What about in your personal life? You said you wouldn't come for work concerns, but do you have other concerns of your own?*
PT: *Well, I'm 46 and haven't been able to have a relationship with a woman that is satisfying and lasting.*
TH: *How is that a problem for you?*
PT: *Well, I'd like to get married and have a family at some point.*
TH: *What's been in the way, do you think?*
PT: *Again, I am demanding and have no patience with people who don't measure up.*

TH: *So you are just as demanding in your personal and romantic relationships with women as you are with employees at work?*

PT: *I guess that's true.*

TH: *And how's that working out?*

PT: *Obviously, it doesn't at some level, but I just can't seem to find someone who really captures my attention. I lose interest – there is always something missing.*

TH: *How old are you now?*

PT: *46.*

TH: *And how long have you been dating?*

PT: *Since high school – around 16.*

TH: *For 30 years you have been searching but found no one who measures up. You are the common denominator here.*

PT: *I guess you could say that.*

When patients have so little motivation to engage in therapy, and fail to see their role in perpetuating the problems they complain about, working with the transference pattern of behavior, in the here and now, proves essential.

C-T Link

TH: *And if we look at the way you interact here with me, we can see the same level of emotional detachment and lack of involvement that you describe elsewhere. You come all this way – an intelligent and successful man – but can't declare an issue of your own to address – as if you are just here because others say so. You don't strike me as someone who generally takes orders from others.*

PT: *That's true, but I've heard this comment that you just made from others.*

TH: *From?*

PT: *The women – they complain that I am distant and uninvolved.*

TH: *Again, you say others make these observations or complaints, and we can see it in operation here. Clearly you are detached and uninvolved – revealing and risking nothing. The question is whether this concerns you.*

PT: *Well if that's part of the problem and you can help with that...*

Rather than experience any internal conflict, this man has played out conflicts regarding closeness with others. Women pursue him and he distances. The therapist was intentional about keeping the focus internal and refusing to get into a battle of wills or interpersonal conflict with him.

TH: *Let's not create a conflict here, between you and me. It's up to you to decide if this is a problem you want to look into and get some help with. You say you'd like to get married and have a family, but you remain distant and remote. Clearly, there is a conflict there – saying one thing and doing another. You focus on others rather than having a deep look within yourself. I wonder if you have ever gotten close to anyone?*

PT: *I'm not really sure that I have. My mother died recently, and I didn't shed a tear. It makes me wonder if I ever loved her.*

TH: *You seem to have created a massive barrier to closeness to others. You feel no pain and sorrow but no love either. What is it like to live like that?*

PT: *Well, maybe I shouldn't say never. I was really in love in my early 20s, but she dumped me.*

Since the defense of detachment was highly syntonic and worked for him in many ways, it took a good deal of time and attention to create a shift in which he started to see (and feel) the cost of this characteristic pattern of behavior. He remembered his first romantic relationship and how devastated he was when the woman he loved left him. She wanted children and he wasn't ready for such a commitment, so she left him. He realized that he had shut down after this experience and sealed his heart, leaving him alone and isolated. He felt grief about the loneliness in his life and began to cry. This seemed to be an important breakthrough and was a hopeful sign, or so it seemed. However, in the next session, his defenses were fortified and the wall he erected to genuine contact proved impenetrable.

PT: *I felt like a real loser yesterday.*

TH: *That sounds like a pretty harsh judgment. How do you understand it?*

PT: *Crying here with you is pretty pathetic. What happened with my girlfriend was so long ago.*

TH: *Again, pretty harsh. I wonder how you are feeling toward me for encouraging you to have a look at those feelings of pain and grief?*

Since his defenses had intensified and he was treating himself in such a harsh and self-critical manner, the possibility that anger toward the therapist was being self-directed was investigated.

PT: *I think you just wanted to get a rise out of me.*

Instead of declaring his feelings toward me, another defense (projection) emerged. Kernberg (1994) has suggested that patients with narcissistic characters often have a borderline level of ego organization. As this man's mask started to crack, his tendency to split and project became evident. It is rare for such patients to be treated rapidly and most need longer term therapy.

TH: *You go to thoughts and judgments – about yourself, and about me – but that doesn't say how you feel.*

PT: *This whole feeling business is so formulaic. Like you go to therapy and cry about your mother.*

Dismissiveness and contempt are common in narcissistic characters and prevent access to feelings buried beneath these defenses. They also create a massive resistance to closeness with the therapist. Both were clearly present in this case and proved unresponsive to a brief therapeutic encounter. Perhaps another therapist or another approach might have been more effective, but research suggests this is a highly treatment-resistant population (Kernberg, 1994).

TH: *There is a real sense of contempt coming up. Clearly you had feelings about having opened up here and revealed some vulnerability. Once again, there is massive shutdown and distancing here with me. Do you recognize this pattern?*

PT: *Look, I came here because I was asked to and am leaving this afternoon. What is the point?*

TH: *Is this what happens in life? You give up? What's the use, if there is no guarantee?*

Try as I might to reestablish some agreement about what we were going to do with our time together, the patient's defenses only got stronger after the breakthrough of feeling in the first session. For patients such as this, who are terrified of vulnerability, opening up in such a rapid fashion with no time for a slower process of working through to take place often backfires. Therapy is not, and cannot be, a one-size-fits-all endeavor. We must assess both the patient's difficulties and their capacity and motivation in order to tailor the treatment to their needs. In this case, the patient had given up on relationships in an effort to maintain his self-esteem.

Summary

In this chapter, we have focused on the two innate drives operating in all human beings – to develop an autonomous sense of self and to attach securely to others. In many cases, our patients have sacrificed one of these innate drives in order to achieve the other. In the end, both suffer. Those who lack a solid sense of self can't be truly open and available to others, while those who sacrifice self for relationships have little to offer. Cases of each compromise were illustrated and examined.

Chapter 8

A Good Goodbye

The last note of a symphony is just as important, if not more so, than the first. Similarly, the proper management of the final phase of therapy often proves crucial for success, especially with patients for whom the theme of loss has been prominent.

In this chapter, we will discuss when, how, and why to terminate therapy, with a special emphasis on the importance of creating a good ending. Sadly, this aspect of treatment is often neglected in training and has received sparse research attention (Barrett, MacGlashan & Clark, 2000; Goldfried, 2002; Greenberg, 2015; Joyce et al., 2007; Wachtel, 2002). That said, most agree that termination should take place once the patient's goals have been achieved.

Generally speaking, the longer and more complex the treatment, the more time and attention must be devoted to the process of ending. That said, patients can receive significant, even life changing help, in a very brief amount of time. They can also experience intense feelings when ending a brief, but very significant treatment. Their gratitude for such help, frequently accompanied by grief about how long they have suffered, and anger at other helpers who have failed them, can be profound. This underscores the fact that length of treatment does not determine its effectiveness, nor its lasting benefit. Given this, it is not a primary consideration in determining when to end. In fact, just such a case finished up yesterday.

A Woman Scorned

A 50-year-old divorced female professional sought help to address anxiety in relationships. Especially since going through a highly contentious divorce, in which she lost a great deal of money (as well as her heart), she was gun shy about committing herself to her current beau – a lovely man who seemed both loving and reliable. Inquiry revealed that her anxiety about emotional closeness was more long standing and pervasive than this presenting concern might suggest. However, only six sessions were required to discover the source of her intense ambivalence about closeness and resolve it.

DOI: 10.4324/9781003197669-8

The patient reported having been molested by an uncle as a child. When she told her parents about the abuse, they did not believe her. Despite their refusal to accept her account of what had happened, they severed ties with that branch of the family, and the patient never saw any of them again. This pattern of rupture without repair was repeated often in her life.

Neither of her parents, both survivors of war, were available for emotional closeness throughout her life (except at her mother's death, when some genuine closeness was experienced). In her adult life, she had experienced significant ruptures and betrayals in friendships and professional relationships, adding to the scar tissue of early attachment traumas. She dealt with her feelings about all this by shutting down and withdrawing. At the same time, she longed for closeness and found a compromised way to relating that shielded her from pain but was ultimately unsatisfying.

We were able to see this same pattern of ambivalence about closeness in her relation to the therapist. While consciously engaged in the process, she was emotionally guarded, laughing over her feelings and avoiding eye contact. As these defenses against closeness were addressed, she was able to drop them in order to face feelings of rage, guilt, pain, and longings for closeness. As a result, she was able to commit to her current partner and move in with him. In addition, she spoke about an emerging sense of herself as confident and empowered.

Having reached her goals, she broached the topic of termination. However, she did so via email, revealing her continued reliance on avoidant strategies. I responded by suggesting we make a final appointment to wrap up the treatment. This final session proved highly significant.

PT: *When I got your message, I realized I was being avoidant. I'm so glad you suggested we meet.*

This opening statement suggested that, with some help, she was easily able to spot her defensive reaction to termination and turn it around. The fact that she expressed appreciation for the therapist's suggestion indicates there may have been an unconscious test involved in her email message (Weiss, 1993). In her past experience, it seemed that others did not want to get close to her and were especially averse to sharing strong feelings. Would the therapist accept her invitation to end without closure or pursue her to say goodbye in person?

TH: *I am too. While we haven't worked together long, it has felt significant. We really have two tasks – to consolidate the work we've done – and to say goodbye.*

PT: (Patient began to laugh and then cry.) *Wow – I didn't expect this. I really do have strong feelings about you and the work we have done together. I felt as if you really understood me and were able to reflect that understanding back to me in a way that was really powerful.*

In addition to experiencing and freely expressing her feelings about ending, consolidating the gains obtained in the therapeutic process was another central task of the final session.

TH: *What is the impact that has had?*

PT: *I really got to understand the family pattern and have an awareness of how I participated – and perpetuated – not getting my needs met in relationships later on. I am much more confident – and courageous – now. I speak up for what I want. I even asked for a raise – and got it!*

TH: *That's great. It sounds as if you recognized your own lack of self-worth and, as you have come to recognize and embrace your own value, you can ask for – and get – more. It's like an upward spiral.*

PT: *Absolutely – from the inside out.*

TH: *And what about in your intimate relationship with your partner – that was really important to look at?*

PT: *I wasn't getting what I want because I didn't ask. Now, I ask and am amazed at how responsive he is!*

TH: *When you are clear in the asking, you get a very clear response.*

PT: *That's for sure. With my fiancé, it's a clear yes. With my Dad, not so much. I hugged him the other day and said, "I love you." He nodded. That is the best he can do. I felt sad but didn't take it personally. In the past I would have withdrawn and just given up, but I realize he has been massively traumatized and just can't do it. It was clear he was touched by my reaching out and that was enough for me.*

TH: *You seem so much more self-defined, and no longer reliant on the other person's behavior to determine where you stand.*

In this case, the patient's difficulties were not just the result of suppressed feelings and wishes, but an excessive reliance on approval and validation from others as well. Consequently, the ability to stand on her own two feet and to be self-validated, even in the presence of disconfirmation from others, was required for healing.

PT: *You're right. I went to a meditation retreat last week and, I don't mean this in a boastful way, but I just realized how special I am. I could feel it and embrace it.*

TH: *You mean really acknowledging the gifts you have to share?*

PT: *Yes, it's not about ego at all, but exists at a more spiritual level.*

TH: *The way you've been made.*

PT: *I just felt it again, the sense that you intuitively get what I'm saying* (laughs and then starts to cry).

TH: *It's been a very meaningful connection and there are clearly a lot of feelings about saying goodbye, especially to someone who has been important to you.*

PT: *It feels like graduating, in a way. It's not that I need you to carry on, but I am sad. Somehow it feels parental.*

Examining feelings about saying goodbye to the therapist triggered feelings and memories of saying goodbye to her mother. The patient went on to recount memories of the last days with her mother, in which there was a quiet but profound sense of closeness. She laid with her in the hospital bed as she slipped away from life. This felt sense of closeness and love in the end was experienced as healing.

TH: *How can we have a good goodbye?*
PT: (Really starts crying.) *I've had horrible endings in my life. It was beyond awful with my ex-husband, and I've been betrayed by friends and colleagues. Of course, there was my uncle who molested me and how my family severed ties after that. I never saw him or any of that side of the family again! And we never talked about it!*
TH: *Does this feel different?*
PT: *Very much so. I am so glad you encouraged me to meet so I can express my appreciation and really say goodbye.*
TH: *There is appreciation and sadness, but no regrets when you speak from your heart.*
PT: *That is so true. Thank you.*
TH: *It has really been a pleasure to work with you and to get to know you in this way.*

While this was a brief treatment, it had proven deeply meaningful to the patient (and therapist!). She had a history of breakdown and rupture with no repair in a number of previous relationships, so endings evoked intense mixed feelings. Initially, she tried to avoid it all by writing an email to end the treatment. When encouraged to come for a final session to complete the process, she was grateful for the opportunity to experience and work through feelings about loss. She had been unaware of how intense her feelings were about ending and was initially surprised by them. We were able to make sense of her experience together and create a good goodbye instead of another ending without closure and completion. This added significantly to the work already accomplished and further solidified the change in her.

From the start, the most effective therapists gain consensus on the nature of the problems to be addressed, as well as the therapeutic goals and the tasks required to reach those goals (Bordin, 1979, 1994). In any depth-oriented psychotherapy, the overarching purpose and goal of treatment includes a resolution to the conflicts responsible for the patient's symptoms and suffering, in order to free them to live authentically and function at their highest level of capacity. In this sense, the end is clear from the start. Malan (Malan & Coughlin Della Selva, 2007) suggested ambitious criteria for termination

– that every symptom and pathological defense be not simply removed but replaced with a healthy alternative. The achievement of these goals becomes the basis upon which we determine when termination should take place.

In addition to reviewing the therapeutic process and consolidating therapeutic gains at termination, the creation of a good goodbye can enhance the benefits accrued during therapy (Davis, 2008). This process was illustrated in the case just reviewed. In contrast, a poor ending can undermine the progress made during treatment and leave an enduring bitter taste in the mouth. Had I simply accepted the patient's suggestion that we end for now, without having a final session, it would have reinforced her avoidance and could well have eroded her budding confidence in being able to create and sustain close and meaningful relationships. Therefore, it is of the utmost importance that what went wrong with endings in the past should go right. To accomplish these ends, the therapist must plan an approach that is suited to each patient and implemented with skill, focused attention, and empathy. Dealing with all the mixed feelings about saying goodbye to someone who has become very important is a central task of the termination phase of therapy.

Needless to say, termination can evoke strong mixed feelings in the therapist, as well as the patient. A keen awareness of our own vulnerabilities around loss is essential, lest we act out our own countertransference during this period of the work. Examples of this include continuing to see patients long after they achieved their goals and/or providing excessive reassurance that the patient can contact us, should the need arise. In contrast, a number of patients have reported that their analysts acted out by suddenly terminating with them unilaterally when the patient expressed concern about the length of treatment or sought out a consultation. In two other recent cases, it was reported that male therapists abruptly terminated treatment after their female patients revealed sexual and romantic feelings for them. Rather than dealing with these feelings and wishes therapeutically, as we would any other set of feelings, they acted out their countertransference. In each case, the patient reported feeling proud of herself for honestly revealing feelings that were difficult to disclose, but intensely distressed about being responded to in such a way that was experienced as harmful.

Feelings to Be Expected at Termination

Most of the literature on termination focuses on grief and mourning as the most striking affect experienced during this time. Early in my career, as a traditional dynamic therapist, the ending of therapy was, in fact, usually a sad affair, in which grief around loss was the prominent feature. Once I started to practice ISTDP, in which treatments were more intense, rapid, and effective, the whole tenor of the termination phase changed dramatically. Much to my surprise and delight, the termination phase of Intensive Short-Term Dynamic Psychotherapy (ISTDP) was often distinctly celebratory. Feelings of deep gratitude for the hard work and devotion of the therapist, as well as genuine pride in themselves for overcoming anxiety and inhibition to become authentically self-expressed, became the order of the day. There were feelings of sadness, for sure, but they seemed to pale in comparison to these more "positive" effects of appreciation, gratitude, pride, and confidence. In my previous practice, as a more traditional dynamic therapist, there was a tendency to be suspicious of positive feelings and to consider those of sadness, disappointment, and rage more genuine and important.

As patients began to express their heartfelt gratitude for partnering with them on a difficult but transformational journey, I was challenged to take in and appreciate the need to receive these sentiments openly. Mutuality and reciprocity are a hallmark of healthy relationships. When a difficult but ultimately freeing process of healing is traversed together, this kind of mutuality is created, sometimes for the first time in the patient's life.

In the early days of my practice, I tended to minimize and even dismiss these positive comments about my contribution to therapeutic success, in favor of attributing all the gains to the patient alone. Over time, I came to realize, especially when I saw this same tendency in my trainee's videotapes, that such deflection was defensive on my part. I started to open up to the appreciation my patients needed and wanted to express for the help they had received. Deep and lasting therapeutic change can only be achieved when there is a true partnership between patient and therapist from beginning to end.

As therapists on the front lines, we can get used to human misery and become anxious and uncomfortable in expressing and receiving loving feelings. Fears of boundary violations can heighten such anxiety. Leigh McCullough (personal communication, 1996) reflected on the fact that love had become a four-letter word in psychotherapy – something we dare not mention. Luckily, I had worked on my own discomfort around receiving appreciation and gratitude for years, in both my personal and professional life, so that I was able to be open to the positive feelings patients wanted to freely express. My ability to do just that was especially vital in the following case, of the *Man with Unexplained Medical Symptoms.*

The Man with Unexplained Medical Symptoms

The phase of inquiry with this patient revealed a pattern of chronic repression of rage toward his tyrannical and sadistic father, resulting in symptoms of depression and a whole host of unexplained medical symptoms. As one of four boys in his family, he was routinely exposed to bullying by his father, something purportedly designed to make him strong. He was considered the "sensitive one" in the family, who was closer to his mother than his father. For this, he incurred the wrath of his father, who taunted him daily about being a "patsy ass" and a "mama's boy." These verbal slurs were accompanied by punching and episodes of having his head dunked in the pool over and over again, so that he would fight back and "become a man." As he described these episodes, he started to tense up and sigh, suggesting that the conflict around his rage toward his father was intensifying.

TH: *How do you feel this rage toward your father?*
PT: *I feel my heart beating faster and sense tension all over.*
TH: *Would you say that is anger or anxiety?*
PT: *I think it's both.*
TH: *This lets us know you are terrified of this rage. You tense up, keep it in, and then where does it go?*
PT: *Clearly it stays inside and creates all these physical symptoms. I am absolutely convinced of that at this point.*

The patient was fully aware of his triangle of conflict – that he is anxious about his rage toward his father and suppressed it in ways that created and perpetuated his symptoms. This cleared the path for pressure to feeling.

TH: *Since you want to be free of these symptoms, which are caused by suppressing this rage, are you willing to let yourself feel this fully?*
PT: *I am willing, but just can't seem to get there.*
TH: *How much of the rage you know you have toward your father are you letting yourself experience right now?*
PT: *I'd say 20%.*

The patient was highly motivated and doing his best to get in touch with this terrifying rage. He was looking right at me and creating no barriers to closeness. Consciously, he wanted to co-operate and free himself to experience this feeling, but unconsciously, he was terrified and resisting that very thing. I wondered if the trigger to his anger was clear and specific enough to allow for mobilization of his rage, as he was referring to a general, lifelong pattern of bullying. Rather than assume resistance was the major culprit, asking for a specific example was the first line of inquiry to be pursued.

TH: *OK. So, if you think about the thing you are most furious with your father about, what would that be?*
PT: (Looking right at me and speaking slowly but deliberately.) *Well…that would have to be …that he murdered my mother and then hung himself… And, I'm the one who found them.*

It was all I could do to stay focused on his experience and proceed with the work, while containing my own response to this horrifying revelation. He continued with details of that tragic day. He had been calling his mother on the phone but, receiving no answer, decided to go to the house and investigate. Upon entering the home, he discovered his mother's slain body on the kitchen floor. Horrified, and concerned that the perpetrator might still be in the house, he ran back to his car and called the police.

The police arrived and found his father hanging in the rafters of the attic. His father had left a note saying that he was so overwhelmed with grief when he came home to discover his wife's murdered body, that he simply couldn't go on. This sent the police on a wild goose chase for a non-existent intruder and split the family in two.

The patient's father was a prominent and beloved figure in the community, idealized by many, including his brothers, none of whom wanted to acknowledge his dark side. Eventually, all the evidence suggested that his father was the murderer. The patient knew this was true, but his brothers clung to the fantasy that some stranger had done it, preserving their idealized image of their father.

The police investigation revealed that his father was a compulsive gambler who was in significant debt. He had been a controlling figure who had never allowed his wife access to their bank accounts. He also tended to gather the mail before she could see it. The police found overdue bills on the floor, near his mother's murdered body. They concluded that she had intercepted the mail, discovered his financial maleficence, and confronted him: causing him to fly into a murderous rage. Then, realizing the gravity of the situation and his predicament, he killed himself.

TH: *As you tell me this, how do you feel the rage inside?*
PT: *Now I feel it. It's an enormous rage – massive energy throughout my body.*
TH: *What would that rage do if it was unleashed on him?*
PT: *I would kill him! Strangle him! No – wait – I don't want that. That's what he did – he killed himself so he wouldn't have to face the music. I'm not going to let him get away with it. I want him on the stand. I want him to have to face what he did. I want him to confess! I want him to spend the rest of his life in jail, suffering for the crime he committed.*

It is an error to assume that all patients have murderous rage buried in their unconscious. While the patient initially felt a murderous impulse toward his father, he reversed course and declared the wish that he stand trial and spend the rest of his life in prison. Not only does this make a kind of logical sense, but a direct one-to-one relationship between this wish to imprison his father for life, and his symptomatic suffering, added meaning and significance to the nature of his difficulties. In fact, he was the one who had been serving this sentence since the perpetuation of his father's crime.

The experience of previously avoided feeling and impulses is necessary but often insufficient to work through the patient's conflict. Making sense of the material that is de-repressed is essential in this process. In this case, the patient had to become aware of the ways in which he had inflicted the sentence meant for his father on himself.

TH: *But who has been serving that sentence? Who has been suffering ever since this happened?*

PT: *Oh my God. I'm the one who has been suffering mentally and physically ever since. I am done with that. He should suffer! He was the bastard who killed my mother! Then, the way he still tried to weasel out of it and play the victim – as if he was a loving husband. Then my brothers sided with him. To this day, they don't want to believe he did it!*

TH: *Sounds like you have feelings toward them too, but let's stick with your father for now.*

In fact, all of the patient's symptoms started after the murder/suicide of his parents. Making links between the repression of his anxiety-laden and guilt-ridden feelings and his symptoms was deeply healing. During the next few sessions, more rage and grief about the murder/suicide was experienced, as well as long simmering rage regarding relentless competition with his brothers. He remembered a particular incident in which they were all kayaking together, when they came upon a sudden drop with rushing white water. He recalled an impulse to push his older brother's kayak over the edge, sending him plummeting to his death. This was followed by a deep sense of guilt. He was able to see how both suppressed rage and guilt about his violent impulses was another factor driving his need to suffer. He decided to commute his own sentence and free himself to fully enjoy his life.

This work was remarkably effective at alleviating all his symptoms. Once he was able to face and experience all of his intense mixed feelings toward family members, the repression of which was causing his symptoms, he was freed up substantially. This symptomatic improvement was accompanied by substantial character change. Now that he had unencumbered access to his anger, longings and desires, he was able to become assertive and go after what he wanted, as well as standing up against oppression at home and at work. His wife and boss were especially responsive to his assertiveness and his relationships improved markedly.

After nearly 30 sessions of intense and, ultimately, satisfying work, we agreed to terminate therapy. Having lost both parents in a highly traumatic fashion, and never having had the chance to say goodbye to them, creating a planned goodbye with me was especially important. The following transcript is of our final session together. Of interest, he emphasized nearly every empirically validated factor associated with positive outcome in psychotherapy.

TH: *Tell me what you're feeling about ending today.*

PT: *A lot of feelings. I can't even put into words the amount of gratitude I have for you. I was crying at my desk today thinking about it. I really have a need to share this with you. First of all, I want to thank you for committing your life to becoming what I consider the equivalent of an elite professional athlete. Clearly you have God given gifts, but you have leveraged that, and you didn't do other things so you could commit yourself and push yourself to continuously evolve and learn. I can't imagine all the hours and, maybe torment, in dealing with all sorts of patients, but sticking with it and getting to the point where you can be so incredibly effective so you can alleviate suffering in the world. It's such a gift of love that you have given. It's a legacy that will affect me, my family, and my kids. Multiply that by all the other patients you treat and therapists you train, and their patients. I feel so lucky to have had you as my therapist…(Quiet connection.)…There is more.*

TH: *Let me just ask you – of course I want to hear everything you have to say – but don't want you to talk over the feelings you are having. Can we take a moment to check in on how you feel this gratitude? You certainly looked moved. How would you describe how you are feeling?*

PT: *Certainly warmth, but also anxiety because it's so important for me to express this to you. I feel a responsibility to you.*

The feelings about ending were understandably loaded, and the patient was noticeably anxious as he began to express them. Rather than let him suffer through this process, attention to the experience of anxiety itself was initiated in order to reduce it.

TH: *Responsibility? Seems to me this is an expression of your generosity of heart, to make sure that I know. So is it just responsibility or wanting to give back in some way?*

PT: *I do, but somehow if feels risky.*

We work therapeutically until the final goodbye. Anxiety suggested some remaining conflict regarding the open sharing of warm feelings, something he had been taunted about ruthlessly throughout his childhood. This needed to be examined in the transference.

TH: *Risk suggests you expected a negative response.*

PT: *Maybe it's a habit because I don't expect a negative response from you. It certainly has been in the past if I was open and vulnerable.*

TH: *That's for sure. Ultimately, it's vulnerable for all of us to open our hearts and to love fully, as all relationships will end, in one way or another, at one time or another. There is something very poignant in this. While you are expressing positive feelings, it seems to be tinged with sadness, is that right?*

PT: *Yes...yes.*

TH: *And yet, in a funny way, it's the ending that triggers the gratitude and prompted you to want to express it – so they are intimately connected. Talking about it seems to have brought the anxiety down.*

Once his anxiety was reduced, he was able to experience and express all his feelings freely.

PT: *Yes. There were other things I wanted to say. Obviously, you are intelligent and educated, and keep yourself open to new ideas, but it's beyond that – it's your integrity and character and your motives that touched me most.*

TH: *What do you mean by that? Are there some examples?*

PT: *Yes, it's obvious that you have strength of character. You didn't need me to be sick. In fact, you have always showed me that my paradigm was false* (that he needed to be passive, compliant and in a needy, one down position to get his needs met). *It took me some time to catch up to that, but you are so solid that you didn't use me for your needs. You do whatever is necessary, whether it's saying something difficult and uncomfortable, for you or for me, and pushing me – whatever is necessary to get the result. My primary experience in sitting here for nearly 30 times is that you... it's like in hockey – you are above your skates – I feel like, when we were really into something important, there was a steely eyed, stare anybody down* (I laughed), *and also the laugh – you are somehow more than just a person. I don't know how to describe it.*

The patient was describing a therapeutic stance that Malan referred to as having "an iron fist in a velvet glove." That combination of strength, courage, warmth, and authenticity seemed to be especially powerful in this case.

TH: *Is it the quality of attention? You're saying you have the sense that I'm not doing this to get my personal needs met, but that my attention is completely focused on you, or how would you?*

PT: *Absolutely, but it's also more than you – not just you. There is something ageless – when we were deep and connected, there was a timeless quality.*

TH: *In that depth of connection there is a timeless quality.*

PT: *I always felt like you could handle anything, and you always did. I could open the cellar door and reveal everything – whether it was a feeling I had stuffed forever, or a memory or a current situation and you never flinched. You looked at me like I was OK. You weren't shocked and you never disapproved. You have that solid core which, combined with everything else, is what made you so effective. I am thinking about all the other therapists I have seen. Most of them were trying to do the right thing, and some were helpful, but generally speaking, most people get into this business because of their own needs and issues. You never required anything of me. You probably know all this, but I thank you for letting me express it fully* (His wife and others in his life tended to be very anxious about and dismissive of his positive, loving feelings.)

TH: *I really appreciate it. It so clearly comes from your heart, and it means a lot to me to hear this. We have both experienced this – this deep connection – and there is almost a sense of the sacred. Are there specific moments that really stood out? I will never forget our first session and certainly other sessions as well.*

PT: *There were a couple of times when you were putting pressure on me to get in touch with some difficult feelings. It was about my mother that was most difficult. You tried the front door, but it was bolted shut. Then, you went off to water some flowers and snuck in the back door. That got me.*

TH: *How did I do that?*

PT: *I don't remember but I was so resistant to looking at the anger toward her. Somehow you took the pressure off, and I could relax. Then, you went fishing – something subtle – that helped me connect to that anger I had never allowed myself to feel before. I don't remember exactly how. You are a pro at picking up cues. I think the biggest thing is your character. I trusted you almost immediately. I sensed that strength in you. I sensed no anxiety in you as we went to these scary places. If it was going on, you hid it.*

Here, the patient spoke of the importance of picking up non-verbal and unconscious clues to guide the process. Timing and pacing were also mentioned, something that must be tailored to the needs and capacities of each patient. All these qualities, in a therapist who is focused and engaged, and who has a method she employs in a flexible but effective manner, seems to foster trust (Wampold et al., 2017). Creating a strong therapeutic alliance involves much more than simply sympathetic or likable, but also highly skilled and competent. Collaboration throughout the journey is essential. Therapy is not something done to the patient but is a collaborative endeavor.

PT: *You have expectations too – of yourself and of me. You hold yourself to a very high standard and work your ass off. You also challenge me to function at my highest level. Excuse the language, but you've got balls!*

Having high standards, pushing ourselves and our patients to obtain outstanding, rather than average results, is another hallmark of high performers who get the best outcomes (Gawande, 2004).

TH: *Can we say courage* (laugh together)*?*

PT: *It was like we were white water rafting* (interesting image, given them memory of he and his brothers in the white water). *At first, you were doing all the rowing, which was OK with you, but you let me know I'd have to grab an oar. You were willing to get wet and dirty and be there with me through all the shit. The great part was to see that our objective was to have me take both oars eventually and navigate on my own.*

TH: *Then I can put up my feet and enjoy the ride. You're right, the goal is for you to develop your full potential. Not simply remove your symptoms but develop your own strength. Would you say that combination of trust, but also, challenge, was important?*

PT: *Absolutely! For me, the risk averse, it was really tough. Without the trust in you, I wouldn't have gone there, and there were times it was excruciating – to face murderous rage toward my father and brothers, for example.*

TH: *That was necessary to get your freedom.*

PT: *If you need to put a sign out there – it would be freedom – that is what you're selling!*

TH: *I'm not sure I knew it was excruciating. Did you let me know that or were you just grinning and bearing it?*

PT: *It took everything I had, and then some, to go there. But having gone there and come through the other side, I learned to trust myself. I'm not sure I connected that until now. I have a much higher level of confidence in myself.*

This point is worth emphasizing. We don't do ourselves or our patients any favors by reducing pressure and taking it easy. Only when we face what we have feared and avoided, can we gain confidence. Confidence only happens after a challenge has been undertaken, not before. When we challenge our patients, we communicate faith and trust in them and their abilities. Working at the patient's highest level of capacity, rather than focusing exclusively on their difficulties, is essential in promoting deep and lasting change.

TH: *That's wonderful because you came in with no confidence in yourself.*

PT: *Now I know there will still be rough times, but I can handle it. Like when I had that eye injury and had to be immobile for days, being isolated and unsure about my vision – I was able to be with myself and all my feelings. I remember just letting myself cry like never before. Also being in touch with how much I love my wife and kids. As soon as I could be upright again, I put on the song, "Blue Ain't Your Color" and grabbed my wife to dance with her. Despite it all, I have a light in me. You really primed me for that – for an injury to be a gift. Thanks for that. I have so much love. The way my love affects my wife is amazing – the softening in her.*

TH: *Just to be able to freely say whatever you need to say. Loss and grief are inevitable, but regrets are optional, if we speak from the heart. We never know when loss will happen, as you well know.*

Of interest, this patient confirmed what research has discovered regarding the qualities associated with the most effective therapists (Wampold et al., 2017). These included a therapist who is skilled and competent, as well as engaged, approachable, and responsive. Being structured but flexible, according to the needs and capacities of the patient, and challenging herself and the patient to work at their highest level of capacity in order to reach ambitious goals, are other defining characteristics of top performers. In addition, superior metacognitive skills, such as working memory and pattern recognition, and high levels of emotional intelligence are other factors associated with the most effective therapists. A review of these factors suggests the need for lifelong learning and development.

In this case, the importance of giving and receiving love, as well as experiencing a sense of the sacred, was emphasized by this (and many other) patient but is rarely discussed in our profession.

The Errant Priest

Many of our patients have had no experience with a positive ending. Facilitating a good and therapeutic ending is especially important in cases in which loss has been a central issue. In the case of the Errant Priest, all his symptoms and difficulties were precipitated by the sudden loss of a beloved mentor. This seemed to trigger long dormant feelings about the loss of his father and grandmother when he was a young child. These losses happened to him. In other words, he had no say in the matter and had no opportunity to say goodbye. It was of great significance that he was the one to broach this topic of ending therapy and had a good deal of input into how and when that would take place.

PT: *I have been thinking it would be good to plan the end of therapy. Maybe we could end in June and meet weekly until then.*

Having the patient initiate a conversation about ending is always best. Rather than simply agreeing or disagreeing with the patient's wish, we must examine the factors associated with the intention to end therapy first.

TH: *What brought this to mind?*

PT: *Something happened. I need help to understand it all, but I realize I don't need you to solve my problems. I feel strong. I don't always understand what's happening at the time, but I'm confident that I will get there. I feel powerful and coherent – more integrated and not splitting and acting out. Even when I am angry, I can handle it and don't behave in an aggressive manner or in a masochistic fashion.*

TH: *Can you tell me more about that change?*

PT: *There is space. I can contain it all. My capacity to feel has expanded.*

TH: *Not just your own feelings, but it seems you are better able to pick up on other's feelings too. You are able to consider their perspective, which was something you were oblivious to in the past.*

PT: *You're right. Now I can connect with myself and others.*

He offered a recent example of a time he felt angry and used it to assert himself constructively.

TH: *That is really different – using anger to take a stand and assert yourself, rather than to destroy either yourself or someone else.*

PT: *Yes, it's different. I am able to stop acting out. This is why I know I will be able to end our treatment.*

TH: *How has this all come together?*

PT: *I may not understand it all but in the past my father, grandmother, and even Victor left me. It was not my decision. You are important to me, but I can decide when it's time to end.*

TH: *When you're ready!*

PT: *Yes, and in dialogue with you. We can come to an agreement.*

TH: *To have a good goodbye.*

PT: *I am sad but also joyful. I feel power that I can tolerate it all. I feel like an adult now. I can choose what to do about my sexuality. It is a sacrifice to choose celibacy. I am free to give it up and own that choice.*

TH: *No longer feeling as if you are being forced and either complying or defying the will of another. You can actively choose to sacrifice something of value for something of greater value.*

PT: *Yes, because I want to be a Priest. I want to do a good job and live with integrity. I am happy about this.*

TH: *This is huge.*

PT: *Even now, when I get a sexual urge, I can have a dialogue with myself. It's my conflict. I won't play it out with others. That conflict will be there, but I can choose how to deal with it. I can also have genuine closeness without sex. Hooking up was a very destructive way to deal with these conflicts. I have mastered this somehow.*

TH: *How do you feel as you tell me this?*

PT: *Extremely joyful.*

Last Session

TH: *Here we are. We have spoken about it for some time, but this is our last session. How are you feeling?*

PT: *Sad, sad. I am sad and feel it all over my body.*

TH: *I am sad too.*

We sat in quiet connection with no need to talk for some time. This, in and of itself, was a big change, as the patient had a tendency earlier in our work to talk compulsively. He was demonstrating a greatly increased capacity to tolerate strong feeling without having to do anything to get rid of or discharge it into action.

PT: *At the same time, it is nice. Like we are in this together. I have changed a lot. I became an adult.*

TH: *And now it's time to go off on your own.*

PT: *I suppose the big change is that I can feel these intense feelings and observe them without having to act them out. I still have the same feelings, longings and wishes as always, but my heart is large and I can contain it all. This is the greatest change. The contact with myself and others is so much greater.*

TH: *Now you can trust yourself.*

PT: *Exactly.* (sitting quietly) *Even now, it's bittersweet – happy and sad. I can allow it and feel it all. When we share it, there is joy. There is really something precious here. You are precious to me.*

TH: *We have almost come back to where we started. It was the loss of Victor that precipitated the problems. You were resisting it, saying it shouldn't have happened. Now you can accept loss and all your feelings about it in such a way that you stay connected to all that was good and previous in the relationship.* (Silence, each of us getting tears in our eyes.)

PT: *Now, I am moved and can see that you are too. This has been so important to me. You invited me to show you my true face. Your face is also true.*

TH: *You are saying that there is something about my authenticity and being real, rather than hiding behind a mask, that has been important?*

PT: *Of course! It was so healing for me – and inspiring. You gave me motivation to be real. You were honest and I could be honest too. Now I can do this outside of here too.*

TH: *We really did this together.* (quiet)

PT: *It's like a prayer between us.*

TH: *It's almost sacred.*

PT: *It is. It is good. I am deeply moved. I have changed and won't turn back. To be open hearted. It is healing. This is a big lesson for me. When there is this genuine connection, there is profound happiness. This is what life is all about.*

Love and loss are flip sides of the same coin. Those who can't grieve can't love. Conversely, by allowing ourselves to feel the pain of loss, we can open our hearts and love more deeply knowing that, even though loss is inevitable, our memories never die. Freud said, "Two hallmarks of a healthy life are the abilities to love and to work."

Summary

In this chapter, we have discussed the prerequisites for creating a good ending to therapy. Doing so consolidates the process of change and further solidifies the gains made. Reviewing the process and elucidating the mechanisms responsible for the both the creation and remediation of symptoms and suffering is necessary. Facing, experiencing, and expressing all the mixed emotions triggered by the ending of therapy is also crucial for success. Three cases were used to illustrate the process. While each therapy differed in length, from six sessions (A Woman Scorned) to 30 sessions (The Man with Unexplained Medical Symptoms), to two years (The Errant Priest), the process involved many of the same elements, including mixed feelings of sadness and joy. The topics of love and a sense of the sacred often arise when the therapy has been truly transformational. This process requires the therapist to be open and receptive to all the patient's feelings (and her own), including those of love and appreciation.

Bibliography

Abbass, A. (2003). The cost-effectiveness of short-term dynamic psychotherapy. *Expert Review of Pharmacoeconomics & Outcomes Research, 3(5)*, 535–539.

Abbass, A. (2015). *Reaching through resistance: Advanced psychotherapy techniques.* Washington, DC: Seven Leaves Press.

Abbass, A., Joffres, M., & Ogrodniczuk, J. (2008). A naturalistic study of intensive short term dynamic psychotherapy trial therapy. *Brief Treatment and Crisis Intervention, 8*, 164–170.

Abbass, A., Kisley, S., & Kroenke, K. (2008). Short-term psychodynamic psychotherapy for somatic disorders. *Psychotherapy and Psychosomatics, 78*, 265–274.

Abbass, A., Kisley, S.R., Town, J.M. Leichsenring, F., Friessen, E., DeMatt, S., Gerber, A., Dekker, J., Rabring, S., Rusalovska, S, Crowe, E. (2014). Short-term psychodynamic psychotherapies for common mental disorders. *The Cochrane Library.* The Cochrane Collaboration. New York: John Wiley.

Abbass, A. & Schubiner, H. (2018). *Hidden from view: A clinician's guide to psychophysiologic disorders.* San Luis Obispo, CA: MindBody Publishing.

Abbass, A., Town, J.M., & Driessen, E. (2012). Intensive short-term dynamic psychotherapy: A systematic review and meta-analysis of outcome research. *Harvard Review of Psychiatry, 20*, 97–108.

Abbass, A., Town, J., Ogrodniczuk, J., Joffres, M., & Lillengren, P. (2017). Intensive short tern dynamic psychotherapy trial therapy effectiveness and the role of "unlocking the unconscious." *Journal of Nervous and Mental Disorders, 205*, 453–457.

Ackerman, S.J. & Hilsenroth, M.J. (2003). A review of therapist characteristics and techniques positively impacting the therapeutic alliance. *Clinical Psychology Review, 23(1)*, 1–33.

Alexander, F. & French, T.M. (1946). *Psychoanalytic therapy.* New York: Ronald Press.

Angus, L., Lewin, J., Boritz, T., Bryntwick, E., Carpenter, N., Watson-Gaze, J., & Greenberg, L. (2012). Constructivist Approach to Assessing Client Change Process in Emotion-Focused Therapy of Depression. *Research in Psychotherapy, 15*, 54–61.

Arieti, S. (1974). *Interpretation of schizophrenia.* New York: Basic Books.

Aron, L. (1991). Working through the past – Working toward the future. *Contemporary Psychoanalysis, 27*, 81–108.

Aspland, H., Llewelyn, S., Hardy, G.E., Barkham, M., & Stiles, W. (2008). Alliance ruptures and rupture resolution in cognitive-behavior therapy: A preliminary task analysis. *Psychotherapy Research, 18*, 699–710.

Baldwin, S.A., Wampold, B.E., & Imel, Z.E. (2007). Untangling the alliance-outcome correlation: Exploring the relative importance of therapist and patient variability in the alliance. *Journal of Consulting and Clinical Psychology, 75(6)*, 842–852.

Balint, M. (1968). *The doctor, his patient and the illness*. 2nd Edition. London: Pitman Paperbacks.

Balint, M., Ornstein, P.H., & Balint, E. (1972). *Focal psychotherapy: An example of applied psychoanalysis*. London: Tavistock.

Bandura, A. (2008). Toward an agentic theory of the self. In H.W. Marsh, R.G. Craven, & D.M. McInerey (Eds). *Self processes, learning and enabling human potential* (pp. 15–45). Greenwich, CT: Information Age Publishers.

Barlow, D.H. (2000). Unraveling the mysteries of anxiety and its disorders from the perspective of emotion theory. *American Psychologist, 55(11)*, 1247–1263.

Barlow, D.H., Farchione, T.J., Fairholme, C.P., & Ellard, K.K. (2011). *Unified protocol for transdiagnostic treatment of emotional disorders*. New York: Oxford University Press.

Barrett, M.S., Chua, W-J., Crits-Christoph, P., Gibbons, M.B., Casiano, D., & Thompson, D. (2008). Early withdrawal from mental health treatment: Implications for psychotherapy practice. *Psychotherapy, 45(2)*, 247–267.

Barrett, J.E., MacGlashan, S., & Clark, A.J. (2000). Risk management and ethical issues regarding termination and abandonment. In L. VandeCreek, & T.L. Jackson (Eds). *Innovations in clinical practice* (pp. 231–246). Sarasota, FL: Professional Resources Press.

Beckstead, D.J., Hatch, A.L., Lambert, M.J., Eggett, D.L., Goates, M.K., & Vermeersch, D.A. (2003). Clinical significance of the Outcome Questionnaire (OQ–45.2). *The Behavior Analyst Today, 4(1)*, 86–97.

Binder, J.L. & Strupp, H.H. (1997). "Negative process": A recurrently discovered and underestimated facet of therapeutic process and outcome in the individual psychotherapy of adults. *Clinical Psychology: Science and Practice, 4(2)*, 121–139.

Blatt, S.J. (2008). *The polarities of experience*. Washington, DC: American Psychological Association.

Blatt, S.J., Auerbach, J.S., & Levy, J.N. (1997). Mental representations in personality development, psychopathology, and the therapeutic process. *Review of General Psychology, 1*, 351–374.

Blatt, S.J., Besser, A., & Ford, R.Q. (2007). Two primary configurations of psychopathology and change in thought disorder in long-term intensive inpatient treatment of seriously disturbed young adults. *The American Journal of Psychiatry, 164(10)*, 1561–1567.

Blatt, S.J. & Luyten, P. (2010). Relatedness and self-definition in normal and disrupted personality development. *Handbook of interpersonal psychology: Theory, research, assessment and Therapeutic interventions*. Horowitz, L.M & Stack, S. (Eds). (pp. 37–56). New York: Wiley.

Blatt, S.J. & Shahar, G. (2004). Stability of the patient-by-treatment interaction in the Menninger Psychotherapy Research Project. *Bulletin of the Menninger Clinic, 68(1)*, 23–38.

Blatt, S.J. & Zuroff, D.C. (2005). Empirical evaluation of the assumptions in identifying evidence based treatments in mental health. *Clinical Psychology Review, 25(4)*, 459–86.

Bordin, E. (1979). The generalizability of the psychoanalytic concept of the working alliance. *Psychotherapy, 16*, 252–260.

Bordin, E. (1994). Theory and research in the therapeutic workshop alliance: New directions. In A.O. Horvath & L.S. Greenberg (Eds). *The working alliance: Theory, research and practice* (pp. 12–37). New York: Wiley.

Bourke, M.E. & Grenyer, B.F.S. (2010). Psychotherapists' response to borderline personality disorder: A core conflictual relationship theme analysis. *Psychotherapy Research, 20(6)*, 680–691.

Bruer, J. & Freud, S. (1985/1995). Studies on hysteria. In J. Strackey (ed). *The standard edition of the complete works of Sigmund Freud* (Vol. 2, xxxii, pp. 1–335). London: Hogarth Press.

Buchheim, A., Viviani, R., Kessler, H., Kachela, H., Cierpka, M., Roth, G. et al. (2012). Changes in prefrontal limbic function in major depression after 15 months of long term psychotherapy. *PLoS One, 7(3)*, e33745. http://doi.org/10.1371/journal.ponme.0033745

Butler, S.F. & Binder, J.L. (1987). Cyclical psychodynamics and the triangle of insight: An integration. *Psychiatry: Interpersonal and Biological Processes, 50(3)*, 218–231.

Castonguay, L., Constantino, J.J, McAleavey, A.A. & Godlfried, M.R. (2010). Therapeutic alliance in CBT. In J.C. Muran & J.P. Barber (eds). *The therapeutic alliance: An evidence based guide to practice* (pp. 150–171). New York: Guilford.

Castonguay, L., Goldfied, M.R., Wiser, S., Raue, P.J., & Hayes, A.M. (1996). Predicting the effect of cognitive therapy for depression: A study of unique and common factors. *Journal of Consulting and Clinical Psychology, 64*, 497–504.

Clark, G.S. & Scharff, D.E. (2014). *Fairbairn and the object relations tradition*. New York: Routledge.

Clemence, A.J., Fowler, J.C., Gottdiener, W., & Krikorian, S. (2011). Microprocess examination of therapeutic immediacy in a dynamic research interview. *Psychotherapy: Process, Research, Practice and Training, 49*, 317–329.

Coughlin, P. (2017). *Maximizing effectiveness in dynamic psychotherapy*. New York: Routledge.

Coughlin Della Selva, P. (1991). The emergence and working through of pre-verbal trauma in short-term dynamic psychotherapy. *International Journal of Short-term Psychotherapy, 6*, 195–216.

Coughlin Della Selva, P. (1992). Achieving character change in ISTDP: How the experience of affect leads to the consolidation of the self. *International Journal of Short-term Psychotherapy, 7*, 73–87.

Coughlin Della Selva, P. (1993). The significance of attachment theory for the practice of intensive short-term dynamic psychotherapy. *International Journal of Short-Term Psychotherapy, 8*, 189–206.

Coughlin Della Selva, P. (1996). *Intensive short-term dynamic psychotherapy: Theory and technique*. New York: Wiley & Sons.

Coughlin Della Selva, P. (2004). *Intensive short-term dynamic psychotherapy: Theory and technique*. London: Karnac Books.

Coughlin Della Selva, P. (2006). Emotional processing in the treatment of psychosomatic disorders. *Journal of Clinical Psychology*, In Session, April. In Session, 62, 539–550.

Coughlin Della Selva, P. & Malan, D. (2007). *Lives transformed: A revolutionary method of dynamic psychotherapy*. London: Karnac.

Coutinho, J., Ribeiro, E., Fernandes, C., Sousa, I., & Safran, J.D. (2014). The development of the therapeutic alliance and the emergence of alliance ruptures. *Anales de Psicologia, 30(3)*, 985–994.

Coutinho, J., Ribeiro, E, Hill, C & Safran, J. (2011). Therapists' and clients' experiences of alliance ruptures: A qualitative study. *Psychotherapy Research, 21*, 525–540.

Craddock, N. & Owen, M.J. (2010). The Kraepelinian dichotomy – Going, going... but still not gone. *British Journal of Psychiatry, 196*, 92–95.

Davanloo, H. (1978). (Ed.) *Basic principles and techniques in short-term dynamic psychotherapy.* Richmond, VA, Victoria: Spectrum Publications.

Davanloo, H. (1979). (Ed.) Techniques of short-term dynamic psychotherapy. *Psychiatric Clinics of North America, 2(1)*, 11–22.

Davanloo, H. (1980). (Ed.) *Short-term dynamic psychotherapy.* Lanham, MD: Jason Aronson Publishers.

Davanloo, H. (1990). *Unlocking the unconscious: Selected papers of Habib Davanloo, MD.* New York: Wiley Publishing Co.

Davanloo, H. (1999). Intensive short-term dynamic psychotherapy–central dynamic sequence: Head-on collision with resistance. *International Journal of Intensive Short-Term Dynamic Psychotherapy, 13(4)*, 263–282.

Davanloo, H. (2000). *Intensive short-term dynamic psychotherapy: Selected papers of Habib Davanloo, MD.* Hoboken, NJ: Wiley Publishing Co.

Davis, D.D. (2008). *Terminating therapy: A professional guide to ending on a positive note.* New York: John Wiley & Sons Inc.

Del Re, A.C., Fluckiger, C., Horvath, A.L., Symonds, D., & Wampold, B.E. (2012). Examining therapist effects in the therapeutic alliance-outcome relationship. *Clinical Psychology Review, 32*, 642–649.

Duncan, B.L., Miller, S.D., Hubble M.A., & Wampold, B.E. (2009). *The heart and soul of change.* 2nd Edition. Washington, DC: American Psychological Association.

Eames, V. & Roth, A. (2000). Patient attachment orientation and early working alliance: A study of patient and therapist reports of alliance quality and ruptures. *Psychotherapy Research, 10*, 421–434.

Ecker, B., Ticic, R., Hully, L. & Neimeyer, R.A. (2012). *Unlocking the emotional brain: Eliminating symptoms at their roots using memory reconsolidation.* New York: Routledge.

Ehrenberg, D. (1974). The intimate edge in therapeutic relatedness. *Contemporary Psychoanalysis, 10*, 423–437.

Ehrenberg, D.B. (2010). Working the "intimate edge". *Contemporary Psychoanalysis, 46*, 126–141.

Elkin, I., Parloff, M.B., Hadley, S.W., & Autry, J.H. (1985). NIMH treatment of depression collaborative research program: Background and research plan. *Archives of General Psychiatry, 42(3)*, 305–316.

Fairbairn, R. (1952). *Psychoanalytic studies of personality.* London: Tavistock Publishing.

Ferenczi, S. (1980). *Further contributions to the theory and technique of psychoanalysis.* New York: Brunner/Mazel.

Fiscalini, J. (1990). On self-actualization and the dynamism of the personal self. *Contemporary Psychoanalysis, 26(4)*, 635–653.

Fosha, D. (2000). *The transforming power of affect: A model for accelerated change.* New York: Basic Books.
Fredrickson, B.L. (2010). The role of positive emotion in positive psychology: The Broaden and build theory of positive emotion. *American Psychologist, 56,* 218–226.
Fredrickson, B.L. (2013). Updated thinking on positivity ratios. *American Psychologist, 68(9),* 814–822.
Frederickson, J. (2012). *Co-creating change: Effective dynamic psychotherapy techniques.* Washington, DC: Seven Leaves Press.
Freud, A. (1936). *The ego and the mechanisms of defence.* London: The Hogarth Press.
Freud, S. (1900). *The interpretation of dreams: The complete and definitive text.* Oxford: Oxford University Press.
Freud, S. (1914). Remembering, repeating, and working through. *Standard Edition: 12,* 145–156. London: Hogarth Press, 1958.
Freud, S. (1917). Mourning and melancholia. In *On the history of the psychoanalytic movement: Papers on metapsychology and other works.* London: The Hogarth Press.
Freud, S. (1930/1961). *Civilization and its discontents.* New York: W.W. Norton.
Freud, S. (1937). Analysis terminable and interminable. *International Journal of Psychoanalysis, 18,* 373–405.
Fromm-Reichmann, F. (1960). *Principles of intensive psychotherapy.* Chicago, IL: University of Chicago Press.
Gawande, A. (2004). The bell curve. *The New Yorker,* December 6, 2004.
Gill, M. (1983). *Analysis of the transference. Volume 1.* New York: International Universities Press.
Gill, M. (1994). *Psychoanalysis in transition.* New York: Routledge.
Giovachini, P. (1975). *Psychoanalysis of character disorders.* Lanham, MD: Jason Aronson, Inc.
Goldfried, M.R. (2002). A cognitive-behavioral perspective on termination. *Journal of Psychotherapy Integration, 12(3),* 364–372.
Gottman, J.M. & DeClaire, J. (2002). *The relationship cure.* New York: Harmony Books.
Greenberg, L. (2015). *Emotion-focused therapy: Coaching clients to work through their feelings.* Washington, DC: American Psychological Association.
Greenberg, L. & Pinsof, W. (1986). (Eds). *Psychotherapeutic process: A research handbook.* New York: Guilford Press.
Grenyer, B.F.S. & Luborsky, L. (1996). Dynamic change in psychotherapy: Mastery of interpersonal conflicts. *Journal Counseling Psychology, 58,* 768–774.
Hansen, N., Lambert, M., & Foreman, E. (2002). The psychotherapy dose-response effect and its implications for treatment delivery services. *Clinical Psychology Science and Practice, 9(3),* 329–343.
Heatherington, L., Angus, L., Constantino, M., Friedlander, M.L., & Messer, S. (2012). Corrective experiences from the clients' perspective. In L. Castonguary & C. Hill (Eds). *Transformation in psychotherapy: Corrective experiences across cognitive, behavioral, humanistic and psychodynamic approaches* (pp. 161–190). Washington, DC: American Psychological Association.
Hill, C.E., Thompson, B.J., Cogar, M.C., & Denman, D.W. (1993). Beneath the surface of long-term therapy: Therapist and client report on their own and each other's covert processes. *Journal of Counseling Psychology, 40(3),* 278–287.

Hoffman, I.Z. (1983). The patient as interpreter of the analyst's experience. *Contemporary Psychoanalysis, 19*, 389–422.

Hoffman, I.Z. (1987). The value of uncertainty in psychoanalytic practice. *Contemporary Psychoanalysis, 23*, 205–214.

Hollon, S.D., Thase, M.E., & Markowitz, J.C. (2002). Treatment and prevention of depression. *Psychological Science in the Public Interest, 3(2)*, 39–77.

Issacson, W. (2011). *Steve jobs: The exclusive biography.* New York: Simon & Schuster.

Johansson, P., Hoegland, P., Amlos, S., Bogwald, K.P., Ulberg, R., Marble, A., & Sorby, O. (2010). The mediating role of insight for long term improvement in psychodynamic psychotherapy. *Journal of Consulting and Clinical Psychology, 78*, 438–448.

Johnson, S.M. (2019). *The practice of emotionally focused couple therapy: Creating connection.* New York: Routledge.

Joyce, A.S., Piper, W.E., Ogrodniczuk, J.S., & Klein, R.H. (2007). Structure of therapy and termination. In A.S. Joyce, W.E. Piper, J.S. Ogrodniczuk, & R.H. Klein (Eds). *Termination in psychotherapy: A psychodynamic model of processes and outcomes* (pp. 97–107). Washington, DC: American Psychological Association.

Kaplowitz, M. J., Safran, J. D., & Muran, J. C. (2011). Impact of therapist emotional intelligence on psychotherapy. *Journal of Nervous and Mental Disease, 1996*, 74–84. http://doi.org/10.1097/NMD

Kasper, L.B., Hill, C.E., & Kivlighan, D.M., Jr. (2008). Therapist immediacy in brief psychotherapy: Case study I. *Psychotherapy: Theory, Research, Practice, Training, 45(3)*, 281–297.

Kavanagh, D.J. (1985). Mood and self-efficacy: Impact of joy and sadness on perceived capabilities. *Cognitive Therapy and Research, 9*, 205–525.

Kernberg, O.F. (1995). *Borderline conditions and pathological narcissism.* New York: Aronson.

Kohut, H. (1966). Forms and transformations of narcissism. *Journal of the American Psychoanalytic Association, 14(2)*, 243–272.

Kohut, H. (1984). *How does analysis cure?* (Ed). A. Goldberg. Chicago, IL: The University of Chicago Press.

Laikin, M., Winston, A., & McCullough, L. (1991). Intensive short-term dynamic psychotherapy. In P. Crits-Christoph & J. P. Barber (Eds). *Handbook of short-term dynamic psychotherapy* (pp.80–109). New York: Basic Books.

Loewald, H. (1960). On the therapeutic action of psychoanalysis. *Journal of Psychoanalysis, 41*, 16–33.

Lukianoff, G. & Haidt, J. (2018). *The coddling of the American mind: How good intentions and bad ideas are setting up a generation for failure.* New York: Penguin Press.

Luyten, P. & Blatt, S. (2011). Psychodynamic approaches to depression: Wither shall we go? *Psychiatry, 74*, 1–3.

Macdougall, A.R. (1952). *Letters of Edna St. Vincent Millay.* New York: Harper.

Maciejewski, P.K., Prigerson, H.G., & Mazure, C.M. (2000). Self efficacy as a mediator between stressful events and depressive symptoms. *British Journal of Psychiatry, 176*, 373–378.

Malan, D. (1963). *A study of brief psychotherapy.* London: Tavistock Publications.

Malan, D. (1976). *The frontiers of brief psychotherapy.* New York: Springer.

Malan, D. (1979). *Individual psychotherapy and the science of psychodynamics.* Oxford: Butterworth-Heinemann.

Malan, D. & Coughlin Della Selva, P. (2007). *Lives transformed.* London: Karnac.

Mann, J. (1991). Time limited psychotherapy. In P. Crits-Christophe & J.B. Barber (Eds). *Handbook of short-term dynamic psychotherapy* (pp. 1–52). New York: Basic Books.

Marmor, J. (1978). *Psychiatry in transition.* New York: Routledge.

Masterson, J. (1990). *Search for the real self: Unmasking the personality disorders of our age.* New York: Free Press.

McAleavey, A.A. & Castonguay, L.G. (2013). Insight as a common and specific impact of psychotherapy: Therapist-reported exploratory, directive and common factor interventions. *Psychotherapy, 51,* 283–294.

McCarthy, K.S. (2009). Specific, common and unintended factors in psychotherapy: Descriptive and correlational approaches to what creates change. *Penn Dissertations, 62.* https://repository.upenn.edu/edissertations/62.

Mergenthaler, E. (2008). Resonating minds: A school-independent theoretical conception and its empirical application to psychotherapeutic processes. *Psychotherapy Research, 18,* 109–126.

Messer, S.B. & McWilliams, N. (2007). Insight in psychodynamic psychotherapy: Theory and assessment. In L.G. Caastonguay & C. Hill (Eds). *Insight in psychotherapy* (pp. 9–29). Washington, DC: American Psychological Association.

Miller, S.D., Chow, D., Wampold, B.E., Hubble, M.A., Re, A.C.D., Maeschalck, C., & Bargmann, S. (2020). To be or not to be (An expert)? Revisiting the role of deliberate practice in improving performance. *High Ability Studies, 31,* 5–15.

Mitchell, S. & Black, M. (1996). *Freud and beyond: A history of modern psychoanalytic thought.* New York: Basic Books.

Muran, J.C., Safran, J.D., & Eubanks-Carter, C. (2010). Developing therapist abilities to negotiate alliance ruptures. In J.C. Muran & J.P. Barber (Eds). *The therapeutic alliance: An evidence- based guide to practice* (pp. 320–340). New York: Guilford Press.

Orlinsky, D.E., Grawe, K., & Parkes, B.K. (1994). Process and outcome in psychotherapy. In A.E. Bergin & S.L. Garfield (Eds). *Handbook of psychotherapy and behavior change.* 4th Edition. (pp. 270–378). New York: Wiley.

Pennebaker, J. (1997). *Opening up: The power of expressing emotions.* 2nd Edition. New York: Guilford.

Piliero, S. (2004). Patients reflect upon their affect-focused, experiential psychotherapy: A retrospective study. *Dissertation Abstracts International. Section B: The Sciences and Engineering, 65,* 2108.

Piper, W.E., Azim, H.F.A., Joyce, A.S., & McCallum, M. (1991). Transference interpretations, therapeutic alliance and outcome in short term individual psychotherapy. *Archives of General Psychiatry, 48,* 946–953.

Raingruber, B. (2000). Being with feelings as a recognition practice: Developing clients' self-understanding. *Perspectives in Psychiatric Care, 36,* 41–50.

Reading, R.A., Safran, J., Origlleri, A.I., & Muran J.C. (2019). Investigating therapist reflective functioning, therapeutic process and outcome. *Psychoanalytic Psychology, 36,* 115–121.

Reich, W (1949). *Character analysis.* 3rd Edition. Bellbrook, OH: Orgone Institute Press.

Rubino, G., Barker, C., Roth, T., & Fearon, P. (2010). Therapist empathy and depth of interpretation in response to potential alliance ruptures: The role of therapist and patient attachment styles. *Psychotherapy Research, 10,* 408–420.

Safran, J.D., Crocker, P. McCain, S., &. Murray, P (1990). Therapeutic alliance rupture as a therapy event for empirical investigation. *Psychotherapy, 27*, 406–458.

Safran, J.D. & Kraus, J. (2014). Alliance ruptures, impasses and enactments: A relational perspective. *Psychotherapy: Theory, Research, Practice, Training, 51*, 381–387.

Safran, J.D. & Muran, J.C. (2000). *Negotiating the therapeutic alliance: A relational treatment guide.* New York: Guilford Press.

Safran, J.D., Muran, J.C., & Eubanks-Carter, C. (2011). Repairing alliance ruptures. *Psychotherapy, 48*, 80–87.

Safran, J.D., Muran, J.C., Samstag, L.W., & Stevens, C. (2002). Repairing alliance ruptures. In J. C. Norcross (Ed.). *Psychotherapy relationships that work: Therapist contributions and responsiveness to patients* (pp. 235–254). Oxford: Oxford University Press.

Samstag, L.W., Muran, J.C., & Safran, J.D. (2004). Defining and identifying alliance ruptures. In D. P. Charman (Ed.). *Core processes in brief psychodynamic psychotherapy: Advancing effective practice* (pp. 187–214). Mahwah, NJ: Lawrence Erlbaum Associates Publishers.

Sarno, J.E. (1991). *Healing back pain: The mind-body connection.* New York: Grand Central Publishing.

Sarno, J.E. (1999). *The mind body prescription.* New York: Warner Books.

Schnarch, D. (1991). *Constructing the sexual crucible.* New York: Norton.

Schubiner, H. & Betzold, M. (2010). *Unlearn your pain.* San Luis Obispo, CA: Mind Body Publishing.

Sedler, M.J. (1983). Freud's concept of working through. *Psychoanalytic Quarterly, 52*, 73–98.

Shedler, J. (2010). The efficacy of psychodynamic psychotherapy. *American Psychologist, 65*, 98–109.

Silberschatz, G. (2005). (Ed.) *Transformative relationships: The control-mastery theory of psychotherapy.* New York: Routledge Co.

Stalikas, A. & Fitzpatrick, M. (1995). Client good moments: An intensive analysis of a single session. *Canadian Journal of counseling, 29*, 160–175.

Stark, M. (1994). *A primer on working with resistance.* Lanham, MD: Jason Aronson.

Stark, M. (2019). *The transformative power of optimal stress: From cursing the darkness to lighting a candle.* International Psychotherapy Institute. freepsychotherapybooks.org.

Strauss, J.L., Hayes, A.M., Johnson, S.L., Newman, C.F., Brown, G.K., Barber, J.P., Laurenceau, J-P., & Beck, A.T. (2006). Early alliance, alliance ruptures, and symptom change in a nonrandomized trial of cognitive therapy for avoidant and obsessive-compulsive personality disorders. *Journal of Consulting and Clinical Psychology, 74(2)*, 337–345.

Strupp, H.H. & Binder, J.L. (1984). *Psychotherapy in a new key.* New York: Basic Books.

Strupp, H.H. & Hadley, S.W. (1979). Specific vs nonspecific factors in psychotherapy. A controlled study of outcome. *Archives of General Psychiatry, 36(10)*, 1125–1136.

Talbot, C., Ostiguy-Pion, R., Painchard, E., Lafrance, C., & Descoteaux, J. (2019). Detecting alliance ruptures: The effect of the therapist's experience, attachment empathy and countertransference management skills. *Research in Psychotherapy: Psychopathology, process and Outcome, 22*, 325.

Tatkin, S. (2012). *Wired for love: How understanding your partner's brain and attachment style can help you defuse conflict and build a secure relationship.* Oakland, CA: New Harbinger Publications.

Town, J.M., Hardy, G.E., McCullough, L., & Stride, C. (2012). Patient affect experiencing following therapist interventions in short-term dynamic psychotherapy. *Psychotherapy Research, 22(2)*, 208–219.

Tronick, E. & Gold, C.M. (2020). *The power of discord.* New York, Boston and London: Little, Brown, Spark.

Valdes, N., Dagnino, P., Kraus, M., Perez, C., Altimir, C., Tomicic, A., et al. (2010). Analysis of verbalized emotions in psychotherapeutic dialog during change episodes. *Psychotherapy Research, 20*, 136–150.

Wachtel, P.L. (1977). *Psychoanalysis and behavior therapy: Toward an integration.* New York: Basic Books.

Wachtel, P. (1993). *Therapeutic Communication: Principles and Effective Practice.* New York: Guildford.

Wachtel, P.L. (2002). Termination of therapy: An effort at integration. *Journal of Psychotherapy Integration, 12(3)*, 373–383.

Wachtel, P.L. (2011). *Therapeutic communication, second edition: Knowing what to say when.* New York: The Guilford Press.

Wachtel, P.L. (2014). *Cyclical psychodynamics and the contextual self.* New York: Routledge.

Wampold, B.E. (2001). *The great psychotherapy debate.* Hillsdale, NJ: Lawrence Erlbaum.

Wampold, B.D., Baldwin, S.A., Holtforth, M.G., & Imel, Z.E. (2017). What characterizes effective therapists. In L.G. Castonguay & C.E. Hill (Eds). *How and why are some therapists better than others: Understand therapist effects* (pp. 37–53). Washington, DC: American Psychological Association.

Wampold, B.E. & Imel, Z.E. (2015). *The great psychotherapy debate.* 2nd Edition. New York: Routledge.

Watson, J.C. (1996). An examination of clients' cognitive-affective processes during the exploration of problematic reactions. *Journal of Consulting and Clinical Psychology, 63*, 459–464.

Weinberger, J. (1995). Common factors are not so common: The common factors dilemma. *Clinical Psychology, 1*, 45–60.

Weiss, J. (1993). *How psychotherapy works: Process and technique.* New York: Guildford Press.

Winnicott, D.W. (1963). *The maturational process and the facilitating environment.* New York: International Universities Press.

Winnicott, D.W. (1992). *Through paediatrics to psycho-analysis: Collected papers.* Levittown, PA: Brunner/Mazel.

Winnicott, D.W. (2005). *Playing and reality.* 2nd Edition. New York: Routledge.

Wolstein, B. (1982). The cornerstone of psychoanalysis: Breuer's enduring contribution. *Contemporary Psychoanalysis, 18*, 291–302.

Wolstein, B. (1985). Self-knowledge through immediate experience: A response to J. D. Nason. *Contemporary Psychoanalysis, 21(4)*, 617–625.

Wolstein, B. (1987). Anxiety and the psychic center of the psychoanalytic self. *Contemporary Psychoanalysis, 23(4)*, 631–658.

Yeomans, F. & Caligor, E. (2016). Narcissistic personality disorder: The treatment challenge. *Psychiatric Psychotherapy, 5a(19)*. https://10.1176/appi.pn.2016.4a13.

Index

Note: *Italic* page numbers refer to figures.

For Product Safety Concerns and Information please contact our EU representative GPSR@taylorandfrancis.com
Taylor & Francis Verlag GmbH, Kaufingerstraße 24, 80331 München, Germany

www.ingramcontent.com/pod-product-compliance
Ingram Content Group UK Ltd.
Pitfield, Milton Keynes, MK11 3LW, UK
UKHW020138200926
475702UK00005B/801
* 9 7 8 1 0 3 2 0 5 4 6 7 4 *